Myths in Emergency Medicine

Volume 2

Daniel G. Ostermayer, MD

McGovern Medical School
University of Texas Health Sciences Center at Houston
Department of Emergency Medicine

Daniel P. Runde MD, MME

University of Iowa Hospitals and Clinics
Carver College of Medicine
Department of Emergency Medicine

Manpreet Singh, MD

Harbor UCLA Medical Center
Department of Emergency Medicine

ASSOCIATE EDITORS

Ryan Pedigo, MD

Harbor UCLA Medical Center
Department of Emergency Medicine

Benjamin L. Cooper, MD

McGovern Medical School
University of Texas Health Sciences Center at Houston
Department of Emergency Medicine

ASSISTANT EDITORS

Tom Fadial, MD

McGovern Medical School
University of Texas Health Sciences Center at Houston
Department of Emergency Medicine

CHAPTER AUTHORS

Matthew Negaard, MD
University of Iowa Hospitals and Clinics
Carver College of Medicine
Department of Emergency Medicine

Ryan M. Huebinger, MD
McGovern Medical School
University of Texas Health Sciences Center at Houston
Department of Emergency Medicine

Alex Grossman, MD
Harbor UCLA Medical Center
Department of Emergency Medicine

Miles R. Maassen, DO
McGovern Medical School
University of Texas Health Sciences Center at Houston
Department of Emergency Medicine

Myths in Emergency Medicine Vol. 2 examines the origin, facts, and misconceptions of many common bedside teachings. These are some of the oldest and most pervasive medical myths. With each topic we discuss the best available evidence to guide clinical care and acknowledge the areas of continued uncertainty. Ironically, disproving a myth may actually create a new myth, but these common tales are filled with many falsehoods. By taking a deep dive into these common myths we hope you will both gain an appreciation for medical history and improve your clinical practice and skepticism. Please perform your own research prior to changing personal clinical practice.

Null Publishing

Null Publishing, an academic publisher, provides tools, resources, and expertise to authors publishing educational texts. Authors retain ownership and control, and choose the desired copyright of their published works, while gaining the flexibility and power of digital publishing.

Acute ulcerative upper gastrointestinal bleeding benefits from proton pump inhibitor administration

Matthew Negaard, Daniel Runde, Daniel G. Ostermayer

The Origins

Peptic and duodenal ulcers account for approximately half of all cases of acute upper gastrointestinal bleeds (AUGIB).[1,2] Hemorrhage cessation and clot formation during an ulcer-related bleed is inhibited by low gastric pH and the already-existing tissue erosion. This environment also increases the risk of rebleeding.[3] Proton pump inhibitors (PPIs) decrease gastric acid secretion and may increase gastric pH in patients with peptic ulcer disease if used chronically. If PPIs can increase gastric pH, then perhaps high bolus and continued infusion during an AUGIB could decrease the coagulopathy and tissue damage that initially caused the bleeding while preventing rebleeding and need for endoscopy.[4–6]

This physiologic reasoning originates from an in vitro study published in 1978 describing inhibition of platelet aggregation and the clotting cascade in environments with a pH < 5.[5] From this initial publication, clinical practice adopted empiric use of H_2-blockers[7] and then PPIs for AUGIBs even if the origin (ulcerative vs variceal) is often unknown in the emergency department.[8]

6

The Facts

A meta-analysis of thirty randomized controlled trials (RCTs) of patients with acute bleeding from both duodenal and gastric ulcers found no difference in re-bleeding, surgery or death from duodenal ulcers and a potentially small reduction in those endpoints for gastric ulcers after high-dose H_2-antagonist administration.[9] PPIs emerged as a pharmacologic alternative due to a few pharmacologic advantages over H_2-antagonists. Patients do not develop tolerance to the gastric acid suppression effects of PPIs[10] (unlike H_2-antagonists)[11] and PPIs produce a greater increase in pH (decline in acidity).[12,13]

Although early publications focused on the effects of PPIs on known gastric or duodenal ulcerative bleeds, a Cochrane review in 2010 evaluated research specific to undifferentiated AUGIBs prior to endoscopy. The review evaluated 6 RCTs and found no difference in mortality (OR 1.12; 95% CI 0.72-1.73), rebleeding (OR 0.81; 95% CI 0.61-1.09), or need for surgery (OR 0.96; 95% CI 0.68-1.35) when comparing PPI to controls. PPI use prior to endoscopy did reduce stigmata of recent hemorrhage (active bleeding, visible clot, or a non-bleeding but visible vessel) during endoscopy (OR 0.67; 95% CI 0.54-0.84) and also reduced endoscopic therapies (epinephrine injection, mechanical hemostasis, or thermal therapy) (11.7% vs 8.6%).[14] The endpoints of recent hemorrhage, visible clot, and endoscopic therapies, however, are highly subjective, not patient-centered, and should not be generalized.

The majority of patients in the Cochrane review originated from two RCTs (Daneshmend, et al. and Lau, et al.).[15,16] Both studies showed no significant differences between the omeprazole group and placebo group in the mean amount of blood transfused, recurrent bleeding, or death at 30 days. Again, the subjective measurement of stigmata of bleeding were reduced. Rebleeding rate and mortality within 30 days were not reduced in patients receiving omeprazole (11% vs 8% [p=0.5]; 8% vs 7% [p=0.8], respectively) [17] Taken together, both trials are negative with respect to patient-centered benefits related to PPI administration.

Given these data, the 2012 American college of Gastroenterology (ACG) guidelines and the 2015 European Society of Gastrointestinal Endoscopy (ESGE) guidelines recommend the use of PPI prior endoscopy in order to decrease the proportion of patients with ulcers with high-risk stigmata and the requirement for endoscopic treatment.[6,18] The National Institute for Health and Care Excellence in the UK, however, does not recommend routine PPI administration prior to endoscopy.[19] The 2018 Asia-Pacific working group consensus on non-variceal upper GI bleeding likewise rejects indiscriminate use of intravenous PPIs in stable patients with suspected AUIGB prior to endoscopy.[20]

The pre-endoscopic evidence sharply contrasts with the post-endoscopic PPI administration data. A placebo-controlled randomized trial from Hong Kong showed that the administration of continuous omeprazole infusion (80 mg intravenous bolus followed by 8 mg/h for 72 h) after endoscopic therapy for bleeding peptic ulcers was superior to placebo in reducing recurrent bleeding, transfusion requirements and hospital stay.[21] A meta-analysis of randomized trials of intravenous PPI therapy (80 mg bolus followed by 8 mg/h continuous infusion) vs. placebo/no treatment for 72 hours after endoscopic therapy of high-risk stigmata revealed a significant reduction in further bleeding (RR=0.40; 95% CI 0.28-0.59), surgery (RR=0.4; 95% CI 0.2-0.7), and mortality (RR=0.4; 95% CI 0.2-0.8).[22] The improvement in mortality was specifically in patients having first undergone successful endoscopic hemostasis.[23]

The Bottom Line

- Pre-endoscopy PPIs have not been shown to improve important clinical outcomes in AUGIB such as blood volume transfused, mortality, or rebleeding.

- Pre-endoscopy PPIs may improve stigmata of bleeding or need for endoscopic therapies.

- Post-endoscopic PPI therapy reduces the risk of recurrent bleeding and transfusion requirements.

HIPAA prevents sharing patient information with a treating physician at another hospital unless the patient signs a medical release

Daniel G. Ostermayer

The Origin

Enacted by the U.S. Congress in 1996, the Health Insurance Portability and Accountability Act (HIPAA) provided protections to ensure patient privacy from insurers. The law put in place measures to combat insurance companies that sought to identify conditions and prior medical care of new or existing patients that might cost the company more than the average patient. The U.S. President and Congress intended to ensure that employees could maintain insurance portability when changing jobs regardless of prior healthcare needs.[24,25] The act defined protected health information (PHI) as data created, stored, received, or transmitted by entities or their business associates governed by HIPAA. Although PHI includes all patient health information relating to physical or mental health conditions, and HIPAA prevents transmission without patient consent, it does so only with relation to insurance companies and their business associates.

This protection has been often misunderstood in relation to the sharing of information across hospitals by physicians involved with a patient's care.[26] Physicians seeking historic information to guide emergent care often meet resistance from outside hospital physicians or staff when requesting faxed records, or verbal discussion of a results, because of fear of "violating HIPAA."[27]

The Facts

HIPAA applies to providers, insurers, and business associates who store health data. HIPAA does not provide any intended barriers to patient care and permits disclosure without patient consent of PHI between providers currently or previously involved in a patient's care. Below is a table listing other situations where an emergency department will likely be asked to disclose PHI without a patient's consent.[25]

PHI disclosures not requiring patient authorization

Quality improvement purposes
Public health reporting
Crime reporting and imminent threat prevention
Child abuse or neglect reporting
Domestic violence, neglect, or abuse reporting
Notification to primary care providers of patient's condition and location
To an organization responsible for providing worker's compensation
To an individual exposed to or at risk for a communicable disease

Disclosures of PHI from one provider to another provider for treatment purposes are permissible without the patient's authorization. The disclosing provider must use professional judgment to determine whether the requested PHI relates to the patient's treatment if being requested for information by another physician. When initiating a request for records from an outside hospital, if the records requested pertain to treatment, HIPAA permits disclosure without patient authorization.[28] The law does not describe the specifics on details required for physicians to prove their identity and relation to the patient when requesting information. Often hospitals have instituted release forms to create a paper trail for auditing and compliance, but not because of HIPAA requirements.

Providers may disclose location and general health status to family members if they identify the patient by name, but not the specifics of care unless the discussion impacts immediate decisions. Additional disclosures of treatment details require patient consent. If the patient is unable to consent, the provider must inform the patient that such disclosures were made to family members as soon as possible. However, for providers involved with current or past care, no such permission or disclosures are required even if discussions span institutions.

The Bottom Line

- Providers can freely exchange information across institutions if the information impacts patient care.

- HIPAA directly addresses storage of data and release in relation to insurers and their business associates, not treating physicians.

- HIPAA attempts to balance individuals' right to control access to their health information against providers' need to exchange information for treatment.

Supine positioning post lumbar puncture decreases the risk of post-lumbar puncture headache

Ryan M. Huebinger

The Origin

In the late 19th century, the lumbar puncture (LP) became a prominent procedure in medicine, primarily as a method of diagnosing neurosyphilis. The rise of the LP was also associated with a common complication, the post-dural-puncture headache (PDPH). The PDPH, originally described in 1898 by Dr. August Bier, involved a pressure-like circumferential headache, occurring post-procedure, and exacerbated with sitting or standing.[29,30]

The pathophysiology of PDPHs involve a slow leak of cerebrospinal fluid (CSF) occurring at the puncture site.[31] Many physicians hypothesized about potential treatments including applying catgut sutures to the puncture site,[32] but given the strong positional nature of the headache, experts historically recommended bedrest as a treatment. Physicians commonly prescribed a period of 24 hours to 3 days of rest post lumbar puncture as both a treatment and prophylaxis for PDPHs.[33,34]

The Facts

In the 1930s, researchers first challenged the need for post-LP bedrest as a preventative measure. Despite results suggesting that bedrest after a lumbar puncture did not alter the rate of PDHP, recommendations persisted as a harmless means of reducing symptoms.[35] In 1981, researchers performed a randomized controlled trial showing that immediate ambulation led to a similar of headaches when compared to 24 hours of bedrest.[36] Further studies have been performed since then, and a Cochrane review from 2016 showed that there is no association between bedrest and rate of PDPH.[37]

PDPHs may occur in in up to 40% of diagnostic LPs,[38] but while bedrest has not been shown to decrease headache duration or occurrence, needle type may have an effect on incidence. Many studies have investigated the use of an atraumatic pencil point needle (Whitacre) compared to a traumatic needle (Quincke). A Cochrane review found that traumatic needle use was associated with a higher risk of PDPH compared to atraumatic needles (RR= 2.14; 95% CI 1.72-2.67). When comparing traumatic needles of various sizes, the review found no difference. Similarly, no difference was found when comparing atraumatic needle sizes.[39] The main effect seems to occur from atraumatic needle use not size differences.

Unfortunately, most LP kits are stocked with traumatic needles and many emergency departments do not have atraumatic needles readily available. If using a traumatic needle, insertion with the bevel parallel to the dural cylinder dramatically reduced the incidence of PDPH.[40] This equates to the needle bevel pointed to the ceiling when performing an LP with the patient in the lateral decubitus position or bevel lateral when the patient sits upright. At the end of the procedure, removing the hollow bore needle without a stylet may create enough negative pressure to suction a strand of arachnoid through the dura. This could create a persistent CSF leak, the presumed mechanism behind PDPH. Therefore, insertion of the stylet prior to removal of the needle at completion of the LP can further decrease PDPH risk.[41]

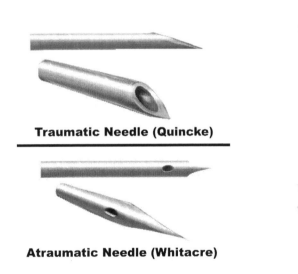

Traumatic Needle (Quincke)

Atraumatic Needle (Whitacre)

Intravenous caffeine ranging from 300 to 500 mg as a multi-hour or multi-day dosing regimen has also been proposed as a means of decreasing headache severity if a PDPH occurs.[42,43] However, many emergency departments and even inpatients units do not regularly stock intravenous caffeine formulations and oral caffeine ingestion has not been studied. In the one randomized

16

trial to show a positive result, the patients were those undergoing spinal anesthesia, not diagnostic lumbar punctures, and the caffeine was administered prophylactically, not in response to a PDPH.[43] Epidural blood patches, with 70-98% treatment success, remain the only therapy for PDPH with robust evidence for support. Unfortunately, blood patches are invasive and have infectious and procedural risks.[38,44] Fortunately, most PDPHs resolve within two weeks with supportive care.[45]

The Bottom Line

- Bed rest after lumbar puncture procedure does not decrease the incidence or severity of PDPHs.

- No quality evidence supports the use of caffeine to improve or shorten symptoms.

- Using a pencil tip (Whitacre) spinal needle is associated with a decreased incidence of PDPHs.

- When using a traumatic needle, position the bevel in parallel to the dural cylinder (towards the ceiling when the patient is in the lateral decubitus position).

- Epidural blood patches and time remain the only therapies supported by quality evidence for PDPH treatment.

Somatostatin analogues (octreotide) improve patient outcomes in acute variceal bleeding

Matthew Negaard, Daniel Runde, Daniel G. Ostermayer

The Origins

Half of patients with cirrhosis develop gastroesophageal varices.[46] Somatostatin is a hormone that reduces portal blood flow and decreases hepatic venous pressure. Octreotide, a somatostatin analogue, has a greater potency and a longer duration of action than somatostatin and increases splanchnic vasoconstriction.[46] In the U.S. octreotide is the most widely available, while vapreotide and natural somatostatin are also used internationally. Physiologically, somatostatin analogues may counteract the pathologic splanchnic vasodilation that occurs in cirrhosis due to the increases in circulating nitric oxide and other vasodilators.[47–49] Major gastrointestinal society guidelines all recommend the use of octreotide for acute variceal bleeding, and administration has become routine for most upper gastrointestinal bleeds in cirrhotic patients.[50–52]

The Facts

The most robust randomized controlled trial (RCT) studied octreotide vs placebo when administered during endoscopy and found no mortality benefit.[53] A Cochrane systematic review in 2008 evaluated the evidence for using any somatostatin analogues in acute esophageal variceal bleeding. The review included 21 RCTs for a total of 2,588 patients comparing somatostatin analogues (vapreotide, octreotide, lanreotide, natural somatostatin) to placebo or no treatment. Patients receiving somatostatin analogues required 0.7 fewer units of transfused red blood cells. Despite decreased transfusion requirements, the study confirmed the original RCT findings of no mortality benefit from somatostatin analogue administration (RR 0.97; 95% CI 0.75-1.25). Also, there was no reduction in rates of re-bleeding (RR 0.84; 95% CI 0.52 to 1.37) when comparing intervention to control groups.[54]

Another meta-analysis often cited in support of octreotide only included eight randomized trials and evaluated the use of octreotide with endoscopic therapy compared to endoscopic therapy alone. Again, no mortality benefit was found but the subjective outcome of "control of hemostasis during endoscopy" was improved in addition to five-day rebleeding rates.[55] These findings garnered support for somatostatins. Although both outcomes are highly subjective, gastroenterologists recommended somatostatin analogues since their use, although not beneficial to mortality, could improve bleeding control during endoscopy.

Neither of the two meta-analyses isolate octreotide-specific studies,[54,55] although it is unlikely that there is a substantial difference between octreotide and other somatostatin analogues with respect to mortality improvements.[56] Also, in all studies, the subjective outcomes of rebleeding and 5-day hemostasis were not predefined outcomes, and their reporting has introduced substantial bias in favor of somatostatin analogue use despite a lack of mortality benefits.[57]

The Bottom Line

- Somatostatin analogues do not reduce mortality in patients with acute gastroesophageal bleeding.

- Somatostatin analogues may decrease the amount of blood transfused in acute variceal bleeding.

- Many studies report an improvement in endoscopic effectiveness (although a subjective outcome) which may contribute to procedural ease.

Ambulance lights and sirens improve the speed and safety of patients arriving at the hospital

Daniel G. Ostermayer

The origin

In 1909, the first motorized ambulance originated in Albany New York with interior domed lamps to illumine the transported patient. Many of these original ambulances were privately owned hearses serving a dual purpose transporting the dead and severely injured. Later model hearses had three lights affixed above the windshield which drivers commonly alternated in a flashing pattern during hospital transport.[58] The perceived speed advantage of lights and sirens during transport— coupled with the eventually common use of police and fire vehicles for emergency medical services (EMS)—led to lights and sirens' being deemed a necessity to ensure quick hospital arrival times. Lights-and-siren transports, especially in dense urban areas, became the default means of battling traffic.[59]

The Facts

A large proportion of EMS personnel work-related injuries and deaths are associated with motor vehicle accidents, many of which occur during lights-and-siren transports. In Colorado from 1989-1997, a retrospective review showed that 74% of EMS collisions resulting in injury occurred during use of lights and sirens.[60] Other U.S. cities have also demonstrated similar increase in risk with lights and siren use.[61] The "wake effect" describes when pedestrian and civilian injuries occur at greater frequency around the areas where EMS units traverse with lights and sirens.[62] The National Association of EMS Physicians, acknowledging these potential harms, released a position statement describing the risks associated with the use of lights and sirens and the need to limit usage.[59]

In 1994, an EMS agency in rural and suburban Pennsylvania implemented a protocol to limit use of lights and siren for non-trauma patients. The change resulted in 92% of patients (sample size 1,625) being safely triaged to non-lights-and-siren transport without adverse effects on their medical conditions or outcomes. Time of transport (mean 18 minutes) did not substantially differ between groups after the protocol change.[63]

In contrast, a convenience sample of ambulance transports in North Carolina within an eight mile radius of the university medical center found a 43.5 second faster transport with lights and sirens to the emergency department. Similarly, another small report found comparable decreases in transport time especially during rush hour (mean 30 seconds).[64] Researchers in Minneapolis, MN, reported on 64 responses over a nine-month period and concluded that responses (time from dispatch to scene) with lights and sirens saved an average of three minutes over non-lights-and-siren responses. Clinical outcomes were not measured and the non-lights-and-siren transports were over longer distances, making direct comparisons difficult to interpret.[65] Similar time savings were reported in a small sample in Syracuse, NY.[66] Although lights and sirens may marginally improve the speed to hospital arrival, clinical benefits have never been demonstrated.

The Bottom Line

- Lights-and-siren transport may provide a small decrease in both response to scene and transport time, although this savings may not have clinical significance.

- Specific traffic patterns, transport distances, and population densities may impact the speed effects of using lights and sirens.

- Lights-and-siren transport is associated with increases in motor vehicle collisions.

Supplemental oxygen should be administered to patients with a STEMI

Matthew Negaard, Daniel Runde

The Origins

Oxygen has historically been included as one of the therapies for patients suffering from a ST-elevation myocardial infarction (STEMI). Theoretically, supplemental oxygen therapy during an acute coronary occlusion could improve myocardial tissue oxygenation. From a physiologic standpoint, if clinicians could increase the percentage of dissolved oxygen in the blood, then cells deprived of perfusion may survive for a longer period of time while the patient awaits percutaneous or thrombolytic therapy.

The Facts

The first major study to question oxygen administration as a default therapy for STEMI patients was published in 1976. The 157 STEMI patients in the trial were randomized (on hospital admission) to six liters/minute of supplemental oxygen or room air for 24 hours. The study found no difference in mortality or incidence of arrhythmias between the groups.[67] Despite this early data, oxygen therapy remained a central part of STEMI treatment for the following decades.

In 2015, the Air Verses Oxygen In Myocardial Infarction (AVOID) investigators published a randomized trial of 638 patients with STEMI on prehospital electrocardiograph (ECG) (441 confirmed with in-hospital ECGs). Patients received eight liters/minute supplemental oxygen vs room air. The group that received supplemental oxygen had an increase in recurrent myocardial infarction (5.5% vs 0.9%; p=0.006) as well as an increase in cardiac arrhythmias (40.4% vs 31.4%; p=0.04). Similar to prior studies, hypoxic patients and those in acute respiratory distress were excluded. At six-month follow-up the supplemental oxygen group had an increase in infarct size based on magnetic resonance imaging (20.3 vs 13.1g; p=0.04).[68] In 2016, a Cochrane Review metanalysis found a pooled relative risk 0.99 for all-cause mortality (95% CI 0.50 - 1.95) using four randomized trials that compared oxygen to room air during the first 24 hours of STEMI care. The Cochrane Review concluded that no evidence supports the use of routine oxygen therapy when caring for patients with an acute myocardial infarction. [69]

Continuing the trend of negative or no benefit, a randomized controlled trial (RCT) in 2017 enrolled 6,629 patients who had STEMI and oxygen saturations greater than 90%, randomizing them to supplemental oxygen (six liters/minute) vs room air. The trial found no difference in mortality between the two groups at 1 year.[70] In 2018, a synthesis of all of the RCTs to date was published in a meta-analysis which, again, demonstrated no benefit of supplemental oxygen in patients with acute myocardial infarctions with respect to in-hospital mortality (OR 1.11; 95% CI 0.69-1.77), 30-day mortality (OR 1.09; 95% CI 0.80-1.50), or size of the myocardial infarction.[71]

The Bottom Line

- Supplemental oxygen offers no benefit for STEMI patients who are not hypoxic or in respiratory distress.

- Excessive oxygen administration may worsen infarct size and myocardial recovery after a STEMI.

- For patients suffering from a STEMI who have oxygen saturations >94%, there appears to be a trend towards harm when providing supplemental oxygen.

Antiemetics prior to morphine administration reduce opioid-associated nausea and vomiting

Daniel G. Ostermayer

The Origin

Many physicians dose prophylactic antiemetics prior to opioid administration when treating acute pain. This practice gained support from the surgical and anesthesia literature describing post-operative nausea and vomiting associated with opioid administration via patient-controlled analgesia (PCA) or epidural analgesia.[72–74] Although the nausea induced effects are more commonly reported in opioid-naïve patients, even those on chronic opioids may experience nausea.[75]

The Facts

Outside of the post-operative literature, no evidence supports the use of antiemetics prior to opioid administration.[76,77] Multiple emergency department studies report a low incidence of nausea and vomiting post opioid administration when treating acute pain. Also, no study has found a significant effect from prophylactic antiemetics in patients without initial nausea who receive an opioid for acute pain.[77,78]

A UK study of emergency department patients receiving morphine were randomized to either prophylactic metoclopramide (10 mg) or placebo.

27

Patients less than 12 years of age, those with existing nausea and vomiting, and those who received prehospital analgesia were excluded. Patients received 0.1 to 0.2 mg/kg of morphine for acute pain in addition to prophylactic metoclopramide or placebo. The overall incidence of nausea and vomiting in the whole study population was 2.7%, (1.6% in the metoclopramide group and 3.7% in the placebo group). No statistical difference was found between groups.[78]

An almost identical study found similar results when randomizing patients to metoclopramide or placebo prior to morphine or meperidine. Seven patients (5.7%) experienced nausea, three in the metoclopramide group and four in the placebo group. One patient (0.8%) had vomiting. None of the differences reached statistical significance.[77] Given a larger sample size in both randomized trials, it is possible that statistically significant results can be found. However, both studies highlight the low incidence and therefore clinically insignificant effect of prophylactic metoclopramide prior to opioids.

Many physicians may still opt to use ondansetron rather than metoclopramide due to the lack of dopaminergic side effects such as akathisia and possibly better nausea prophylaxis.[74] However, ondansetron carries its own potential adverse effects, especially with QT prolongation in patients with cardiovascular disease.[79] Even if ondansetron has fewer adverse effects, with an incidence of nausea of 5% or less post opioid administration, prophylaxis for a rare adverse effect is unwarranted.[77] Additionally, ondansetron was shown to be ineffective in preventing opioid-induced nausea or vomiting. [80] Instead, physicians should wait and reevaluate patients for nausea after administering opioids.

The Bottom Line

- Opioid-induced nausea and vomiting in emergency department patients is uncommon.

- Administration of metoclopramide or ondansetron prior to opioid administration does not produce a clinically meaningful reduction in nausea and vomiting.

Oseltamivir benefits patients with acute influenza

Matthew Negaard, Daniel Runde, Daniel G. Ostermayer

The Origins

The Centers for Disease Control and Prevention (CDC) has recommended the use of the drug oseltamivir (Tamiflu) for acute influenza treatment. Oseltamivir, a neuraminidase inhibitor, impedes viral cell release from infected cells, thereby limiting the overall influenza viral load.[81] Neuraminidase inhibitors, compared to the prior generation of M2 channel inhibitors (amantadine and rimantadine), decrease influenza A and B viral replication. The therapy, first approved for treatment of influenza in 1999, was thought to limit spread of influenza, reduce the risk of respiratory complications, decrease hospitalizations, and reduce symptom duration.[82–86]

The Facts

Although oseltamivir has garnered controversy due to issues with availability of industry-funded study data for inclusion in meta-analyses, much of the debate centers around potential benefits and risks of harm.[82] The first published randomized controlled trial (RCT) conducted on healthy patients with influenza symptoms of onset less than 36 hours found a symptom reduction 30 hours. The authors also claimed that the antiviral drug might decrease the frequency of complications in high-risk populations, but these secondary extrapolations were not directly studied. The second RCT published in 2000, with similar enrollment to the first trial, found a similar 30-hour reduction in symptoms.[87,88] These two trials formed the basis for influenza pandemic preparedness in the form of oseltamivir stockpiling supported by the World Health Organization (WHO).

In a WHO-funded analysis, 74 observational studies were pooled, and it was concluded that oral oseltamivir might reduce mortality, hospitalization, and duration of symptoms compared to no treatment, but generalizability was limited due to confounding, selection, reporting, and publication bias.[86] An industry funded meta-analysis of patient-level data collected during the H1N1 2009 pandemic concluded that the greatest likelihood of mortality reduction was found when treatment was initiated within two days of symptom onset.[85]

In 2014, the Cochrane Review found a mean reduction in duration of symptoms of 16.8 hours (95% CI 8.4 to 25.1 hours, $P < 0.0001$). There were no findings to support prior claims of reduced hospital admissions or prevention of post-influenza pneumonia. Also, no evidence suggests that oseltamivir or other neuraminidase inhibitors such as zanamivir reduced person-to-person spread of influenza.[89]

In 2015, the Lancet published a meta-analysis using the same data as the Cochrane Review. In their intentionto-treat analysis, they found fewer lower respiratory tract complications requiring antibiotics (RR 0.56; 95% CI 0.42-0.75, p=0.0001) and fewer hospital admissions (RR 0·37; 95% CI 0·17-0·81; p=0·013). Similar to the Cochrane Review, the authors found that oseltamivir reduced the duration of symptoms by 25 hours, but common adverse effects included nausea (RR 1·60; 95% CI 1·29-1·99; p<0·0001) and vomiting (RR 2·43; 95% CI 1·83-3·23; p<0·0001).[90]

While there certainly is literature supporting antiviral use, data also suggests the possibility of significant psychiatric and gastrointestinal adverse events, particularly in the pediatric population. Currently, Japan requires a package insert warning against use of the drug in pediatric patients.[82,89,91–94] Specifically, the Cochrane Review reported numbers needed to harm (NNH) for the most common adverse effect of nausea (NNH=22) and vomiting (NNH = 25) that may temper the benefits of influenza symptom reduction. Other less common effects include neuropsychiatric events (NNH = 94), headaches (NNH = 32), and renal insufficiency (NNH = 150).[89]

Although much of the industry-sponsored publications and meta-analyses find more favorable results than non-industry funded research,[95] the most recent non-industry, publicly funded trial supports the findings of prior research. An open-label, multicenter randomized trial of 3,266 patients greater than one year old presenting with influenza-like illness in a primary care setting were randomized to oseltamivir or usual supportive care. Across all subgroups the mean number of sick days was 6.7 with no treatment and 5.7 with oseltamivir. There was no difference in any of the objective secondary outcomes such as hospital admissions or repeat clinic visits. Nausea and vomiting occurred more frequently with oseltamivir: 21% vs 16%.[96]

The Bottom Line

- Oseltamivir, if started within 48 hours of initial influenza symptoms, can shorten symptoms by about one day.

- Common side effects of oseltamivir include nausea, vomiting, and neuropsychiatric symptoms (especially in children), which should be weighed against the benefit of symptom reduction.

- Oseltamivir does not have profound effects on mortality for healthy or unhealthy adults and does not substantially reduce person-to-person transmission.

Nasogastric lavage can diagnosis an acute upper gastrointestinal bleed in patients without hematemesis

Matthew Negaard, Daniel Runde, Daniel G. Ostermayer

The Origins

Patients presenting to emergency departments with gastrointestinal (GI) bleeding require efficient diagnosis and treatment. A large branch in the decision tree for emergency medicine providers is determining if the bleed is an upper or lower GI bleed, especially in the absence of obvious hematemesis. Nasogastric (NG) lavage has been proposed as a mechanism to evaluate for an upper GI bleeding source and triage acuity. Multiple GI society guidelines and consensus publications have recommended nasogastric lavage as a means of triaging non-variceal bleeding patients to more emergent endoscopy.[18,97,98]

The Facts

A single-center, retrospective cohort study in 2012 suggested that NG lavage with findings of black or coffee-ground gastric contents has a positive likelihood ratio (LR+) of 9.6 for an upper GI bleed, which is promising.[99] However, additional studies of larger samples have not replicated such promising conclusions. A review article in 2010 evaluated three studies which compared NG lavage to endoscopy for the diagnosis of an upper GI bleed. NG lavage was poorly predictive (specificity 54-91%, LR+ 1.4-4.7; sensitivity 42-84%, LR−, 0.2-0.65).[100–103] The negative likelihood ratio makes this test poor at ruling out a GI bleed and the positive likelihood ratio make the test poor at ruling in the condition. Also, patients without hematemesis, but with frank melena, already have a finding that is concerning for a GI bleed, and most likely require endoscopy (with or without colonoscopy) to localize the bleeding source, regardless of NG lavage results.

Other studies have evaluated whether NG lavage improves stomach visualization during endoscopy, since placement could assist with endoscopy success. Unfortunately, when compared to erythromycin infusion, NG lavage did not provide improved endoscopic conditions.[104] Additionally, NG lavage does not improve clinical outcomes such as hospital length of stay, need for surgery, or blood transfusions.[105]

NG lavage is associated with deleterious events. It is consistently rated by patients as one of the most painful procedures in the emergency department.[101] Additionally, complications of NG tube placement may be as great as 0.8% with notable adverse events including thoracic placement causing pneumothorax, vascular penetration, esophageal perforation, and tube breakage. Although difficult to quantify from published studies, placement to help rule in or rule out an upper bleeding source could cause additional unnecessary delays. This could be especially problematic for patient care when upper and/or lower enteral visualization is the priority.

The Bottom Line

- NG lavage has poor diagnostic characteristics for ruling in or ruling out an upper GI bleed.

- The procedure is poorly tolerated and carries complications that cause significant harm.

All D-dimer assays are the same

Daniel G. Ostermayer

The Origin

D-dimer assays detect breakdown of the fibrin chains that compose an acute or chronic thrombus.[106] The body's attempt to degrade a thrombus serves as the basis for the assays deployed for acute thrombus detection. These assays' clinical usefulness as a rule-out test requires extremely high sensitivity and negative predictive values. Modern D-dimer tests, which include enzyme-linked immunoassays (ELISA), latex agglutination (qualitative), photometric immunoassays, whole blood (SimpliRED®), and membrane-based immunofiltration assays, have various reference ranges and reporting units, making interpretation non-standard and difficult.[107] Only latex-enhanced immunoturbidimetric and immunofiltration assays (quantitative assays) are fast and sensitive enough for emergency department use.

The Facts

Although the traditional ELISA test still serves as the gold standard for quantitative D-dimer testing,[108] the test requires greater time to perform and is less often used in emergency departments since the introduction of faster immunoassays. Older qualitative latex agglutination assays are not accurate and should not be used for making treatment decisions in patients with suspected pulmonary embolism (PE) or deep venous thrombosis (DVT).[109-111]

The brand and type of assay, however, is not often visible to the clinician. For clinical decision pathways such as age-adjusted D-dimer testing for PE or DVT,[112-114] only a few assays have been used in derivation and validation studies. In addition, D-dimer test results can be reported as D-dimer units (DDU) or fibrinogen-equivalent units (FEU), further complicating interpretation when used for clinical pathways.

For age-adjusted decision making, the original PE derivation study used a rapid ELISA Assay (Vidas®)[112] with validation studies finding similar performance with rapid quantitative latex immunoassays (STA®-Liatest®, MDA®, Tinaquant®, and Innovance®).[113,114] Since immunoassays vary in sensitivity and specificity, providers should only use the previously validated manufacturers in age-adjusted decision making. For non-age adjusted rule-outs, other assays are acceptable.

In addition to manufacturer variability, laboratories may report results with differing types and magnitudes of units. Most laboratories, and thus most published studies, report D-dimer in fibrinogen equivalent units (FEUs). The common cutoff for this test is 500 μg/L. Some laboratories use assays that report D-dimer units (DDU) where the cutoff is commonly set at 230 ng/ml. Thus, 2 DDU (ng/mL) equals 1 FEUs (μg/L). The magnitude of the units may also vary (ng/mL, µg/mL, µg/L) making conversion confusing and requiring special attention.

The Bottom Line

- Age-adjusted D-dimer rule-outs for DVT and PE should only use validated immunoassays.

- Age-adjusted D-dimer rule-outs for DVT and PE utilize FEUs not DDU as the unit of calculation.

- 2 DDU (ng/mL) equals 1 FEUs (µg/L).

An elevated D-dimer mandates a CTA to rule out a pulmonary embolism

Alex Grossman, Manpreet Singh, Daniel G. Ostermayer

The Origin

Current guidelines and clinical practice for ruling out pulmonary embolism (PE) in moderate- to low-risk patients recommend first obtaining a quantitative D-dimer as a means of avoiding pulmonary imaging.[115,116] Using a standardized D-dimer cut-off of 500 FEU μg/L (see previous chapter for D-dimer testing), a negative D-dimer can essentially rule out pulmonary embolism for moderate- to low-risk patients with a reported sensitivity of ≥95%.[117] A positive D-dimer, however, due to poor specificity, requires additional testing to rule in acute thrombosis. This can include either the gold standard CT pulmonary angiography or a ventilation perfusion scan.

The Facts

D-dimer, a non-specific test,[118] elevates in many non-thrombotic conditions that cause systemic inflammation. Common causes of D-dimer elevations include immobility, recent surgery, pregnancy, cocaine abuse, systemic lupus erythematosus, sickle cell disease, malignancy, hemodialysis, and hemoptysis. Importantly, D-dimer levels also increase with age.[119] The 500 FEU μg/L cutoff achieves a high sensitivity at the cost of very low specificity (ranging from 30-50%) that diminishes with advancing age.[120] In an attempt to improve specificity at the cost of a small decrease in sensitivity, age adjusted D-dimer protocols have allowed for avoidance of default imaging in patients with elevated D-dimers.

An age-adjusted D-dimer increases the positive threshold for patients older than 50 years (age [years] x 10 FEU μg/L). For example, a 70-year-old patient would have a new age-adjusted cutoff of 700 FEU μg/L (70 x 10 FEU μg/L). Increasing the positive threshold in fibrinogen equivalent units impacts sensitivity to a small degree while improving specificity and decreasing overall pulmonary imaging. In a retrospective study of 31,094 patients 50 years of age or older, the age-adjusted D-dimer had a sensitivity of 92.9% with a negative predictive value of 99.8%. The 500 FEU μg/L traditional threshold carried a 98% sensitivity and negative predictive value of 99.9%.[121]

The ADJUST-PE study evaluated use of age-adjusted D-dimers prospectively in patients presenting to the emergency department with suspected PE. Patients were risk stratified using either Geneva or Wells scoring followed by a high-sensitivity D-dimer in non-high-risk patients. The primary outcome of missed PE on 3-month follow-up occurred in 0.3% of the age adjusted patients, 0.5% of the patients with D-dimer greater than age adjustment cutoff, and 0.1% in the group with D-dimer below the 500 FEU μg/L cutoff. Notably, the use of the age-adjusted D-dimer had the greatest impact in reducing CT scans in the population aged >75 years. with a 0% miss-rate.[122]

Since this validation, multiple other studies have demonstrated that an age-adjusted D-dimer can safely rule out pulmonary embolism in non-high-risk patients >50 years old.[114,123,124] Using an age adjusted D-dimer in clinical practice can decrease sensitivity by as much as 5% but increase specificity by a similar percentage.[121,125,126] The YEARS algorithm even more bluntly raises the D-dimer FEU threshold to 1000 ng/mL (equivalent to 1000 μg/L) if none of the high-risk criteria are present (1. clinical signs of deep venous thrombosis, 2. hemoptysis, 3. PE most likely diagnosis). Using this non-age-adjusted D-dimer threshold increase led to fewer CT scans and no substantial increase in PE misses.[127]

The Bottom Line

- Increasing the D-dimer cutoff in patients over age 50 years can decrease CTA evaluations and also increase the number of patients safely ruled-out for PE/DVT

- Use of the age-adjusted D-dimer is not appropriate for patients who are high-risk based on clinical gestalt or clinical prediction scores (Wells score or Geneva score)

Blood pressure elevations causes acute headaches

Daniel G. Ostermayer

The Origin

Frequently, patients present to the emergency department complaining of a headache, which they attribute to an elevation in blood pressure. In 1913, Dr. Theodore Janeway published a large case series of private patients with acute headaches and associated hypertension. He described the hypertensive headache as a non-migrainous headache worse upon wakening and resolving as the morning progressed.[128] The study attempted to describe causation but unfortunately given the case-series could only present a possible association between patients in acute pain and those with an elevated systolic blood pressure.[129]

The Facts

Since the original publication, multiple physiologic and population-based studies have attempted to reproduce the direct association between acute pain and elevated blood pressure without success.[130] The most conclusive evidence against blood pressure causing acute headaches originates from a large epidemiologic study. This 11-year prospective study in Norway enrolled 22,685 adults without a history of frequent or recurrent headaches and followed patients for 11 years. The study found no association between blood pressure and headaches. In fact, elevated systolic blood pressure at baseline was associated with low headache prevalence irrespective of blood pressure medication compliance. This study supported the findings of multiple prior small epidemiologic cross-sectional and prospective studies that demonstrated no association between headaches and systolic or diastolic blood pressure.[131–136]

The inverse relationship found in the Norwegian cross-sectional between blood pressure and headaches may be explained by the lesser-known *hypertension associated hypoalgesia* response. Although incompletely understood, evidence in animals and humans suggest that persistent hypertension alters pain response and may increase the threshold to perceived pain, especially headaches.[137]

Of note, many painful intracranial conditions can elevate blood pressure, such as hemorrhage, migraines, posterior reversible encephalopathy syndrome (PRES); all cause other signs and symptoms specific to each condition. These diseases each carry unique findings such as neurologic deficits, encephalopathy, auras, to name a few that make their diagnosis distinct from isolated hypertension. Although accompanied by hypertension, these conditions require targeted treatment irrespective of the blood pressure (with the exception of MRI-confirmed PRES syndrome).[138]

Although hypertension in isolation most likely does not contribute to acute headache, many patients may experience "withdrawal" symptoms from their antihypertensives after missing a few doses or even daily before their first scheduled dose. This creates the association between hypertension and headache as blood pressure spikes after drug cessation or missed doses. Many antihypertensives such as β-blockers and clonidine can produce tachycardia, headache, nausea, and feelings of nervousness 36 to 72 hours after cessation of the drug.[139] Although the patient may attribute the headache to an increase in blood pressure, the cause may actually be abrupt cessation or irregular adherence with the antihypertensive.

The Bottom Line

- Multiple epidemiologic studies have shown no positive association between elevated blood pressure and non-migrainous headaches.

- Acute pain frequently elevates blood pressure and may be a response to the headache rather than the cause.

- Antihypertensive withdrawal symptoms can include headaches and rebound hypertension.

Group A strep pharyngitis requires treatment with penicillin

Alex Grossman, Manpreet Singh, Daniel G. Ostermayer

The Origin

Most pharyngitis results from viral causes and the U.S. Centers for Disease Control and Prevention (CDC) estimates that Group A streptococcus (GAS) may cause 20-30% of cases in children and 5-15% of cases in adults.[140] In patients with clinical features suggestive of GAS, the CDC and Infectious Disease Society of America (IDSA) recommends throat swabbing for GAS testing as clinical features alone cannot reliably distinguish between viral and bacterial causes. Only if a patient has a positive test (either rapid strep or a subsequent throat culture) should treatment be initiated. Treatment of GAS can reduce suppurative complications (i.e. abscess formation), shorten the duration of symptoms, decrease transmission, and, most importantly, prevent acute rheumatic fever (ARF).[140]

The Facts

Though both the CDC and IDSA recommend treatment of confirmed GAS with penicillin-based antibiotic therapy, numerous studies have called into question the benefit of antibiotics. Evidence regarding its main proposed benefit, prevention of acute rheumatic fever (ARF), is limited and based upon studies from the 1950s in young military recruits at Warren Air Force Base.[141,142] Though these studies found a 0.3-3% reduction in ARF with antibiotic therapy, these studies were of poor methodological quality and the applicability of these findings to today's population is limited.

In industrialized countries, the incidence of rheumatic fever has steadily decreased and is now exceptionally low, thought in large part to be due to improved sanitation and possibly shifting GAS serotypes. Epidemiologists also speculate that the widespread use of antibiotic treatment for GAS also may have contributed to this reduction.[143]

A Cochrane review comparing antibiotic to placebo for treatment of GAS infection found 1.7 out of 100 placebo participants developed ARF. However, this only occurred in trials before 1961; no cases were reported in placebo-treated participants in later trials.[144]

Given that the risks of antibiotic therapy, namely diarrheal illness (including *C. difficile* colitis)[145,146] and allergic reactions, are far more common than the risk of acute rheumatic fever in industrialized countries, the potential for harm may exceed any ARF prevention effect when treating GAS pharyngitis with antibiotic therapy. This is particularly true with treatment of adults, as rheumatic fever is almost entirely exclusive to children. It is important to note, however, that these principles do not apply to patients from non-industrialized countries or areas where substantial risk of ARF remains endemic.[147]

Building on the skepticism around ARF prevention, several European guidelines stopped recommending antibiotic therapy for streptococcal pharyngitis as it is considered to be a self-limiting disease.[148] Based upon current epidemiological data, the number needed to treat (NNT) to prevent one case of rheumatic fever may be as great as 2 million patients. Likewise, with low suppurative complications rates (approximately 1%)[149] the NNT to prevent one acute otitis media or peritonsillar abscesses is difficult to accurately estimate.[150,144]

The Bottom Line

- In industrialized countries, the incidence of rheumatic heart disease following streptococcal pharyngitis is exceptionally low; millions of people need to be treated with antibiotics in order to prevent one case of rheumatic heart disease.

- The risks of antibiotics most likely outweigh the risk of ARF in industrialized countries.

- In non-industrialized countries, rheumatic fever is still a major public health concern, therefore patients from these endemic areas should continue to be treated.

- Suppurative complications are increasingly rare with a large number needed to treat, often exceeding the adverse events rate from antibiotic use.

Morphine for patients with pulmonary edema

Matthew Negaard, Daniel Runde, Daniel G. Ostermayer

The Origins

Patients with acute pulmonary edema presenting in acute respiratory distress require therapies that improve work of breathing while addressing the underlying pathophysiology by reducing cardiac preload and afterload.[151] Pharmacologic treatments that perform these functions and relieve pain and anxiety may offer greater clinical efficacy. This reasoning first gave rise to the use of morphine as an ancillary treatment for acute pulmonary edema.

Morphine as a treatment for acute pulmonary edema originated from a canine study in 1966. The investigators concluded that in 18 dogs, morphine reduced pulmonary edema due to increased vessel capacitance.[152] In 1976, a case series of 13 patients with mild pulmonary edema demonstrated improved clinical symptoms after administration of 0.1 mg/kg of morphine. The authors hypothesized it was due to vasodilatory properties or central nervous system effects (decreasing the sensation of dyspnea).[153]

The Facts

Throughout the 1980's and 1990's, several studies began to question if vasodilation was truly responsible for the perceived clinical improvement in patients after morphine administration.[154] In a non-randomized pre-hospital study in 1987, 57 patients with presumed pulmonary edema received nitroglycerin, furosemide, and morphine in various combinations. The small study found that nitroglycerin improved respiratory distress and overall symptoms in the patients with pulmonary edema, while morphine with or without furosemide offered significantly less symptomatic relief.[155] This study was foundational in its critique against morphine as a safe and effective treatment for acute pulmonary edema.

Several retrospective studies provide evidence against morphine's use in acute pulmonary edema. In 1999, a retrospective chart review of 181 patients with acute pulmonary edema concluded that morphine administration was associated with higher rates of intensive care unit (ICU) admission (OR 3.09) and endotracheal intubation (OR 5.04).[156] The Acute Decompensated Heart Failure National Registry (ADHERE) trial analyzed over 147,000 patients admitted to hospitals for acute decompensated heart failure and found that of the patients analyzed, 14% received morphine. Those who received morphine were more likely to require mechanical ventilation (15.4% vs 2.8%, NNH = 8), had longer median hospitalizations (5.6 vs 4.2

days), greater higher rate of ICU admissions (38.7% vs 14.4%, NNH = 5), and had greater mortality (13.0% vs 2.4%, NNH = 10).[157]

In 2017, researchers used the Epidemiology of Acute Heart Failure in Emergency Department (EAHFE) registry to perform a propensity-score-matched analysis of 275 pairs of patients who received morphine vs those who did not and found an increase in 30-day mortality for those that received morphine (HR 1.66). However, there was no statistical difference between the groups in terms of in-hospital mortality or hospital length of stay.[158]

These studies show an association between morphine administration and worse outcomes in patients with acute pulmonary edema when compared to preload-reducing therapies such as nitrates. Although these studies do not prove causation, the current evidence suggests greater effectiveness of preload reduction using nitrates,[159] and clinicians who rely on morphine as primary or adjunctive therapy for acute pulmonary edema should reconsider their clinical practice.

The Bottom Line

- Early evidence for morphine as an effective vasodilatory agent for acute pulmonary edema was weak.

- Morphine administration to patients with acute pulmonary edema is associated with increased mortality, increased ICU admissions, and increased need for endotracheal intubation.

* More effective vasodilatory agents such as nitrates remain the mainstay of treatment for patients in acute pulmonary edema requiring preload reduction.

Lidocaine administered prior to RSI prevents ICP elevation in patients with TBI

Daniel G. Ostermayer

The origin

During intubation, manipulation of the airway can cause catecholamine release, which can increase blood pressure and cause a transient elevation of intracranial pressure (ICP).[160,161] The administration of intravenous lidocaine prior to rapid sequence intubation (RSI) was believed to blunt transient increases in intracranial pressure from systolic blood pressure fluctuations. Physiologically, intravenous lidocaine was hypothesized to decrease the likelihood of induced ICP elevations by decreasing the cough reflex and the catecholamine release that could occur during laryngeal manipulation or suctioning.[162] The dosing of 1.5 mg/kg was given two to three minutes prior to intubation.[163,164]

The Facts

The role of intravenous lidocaine in decreasing ICP elevations during RSI is extrapolated from studies examining the effect of lidocaine on cough suppression,[163–165] endotracheal suctioning,[166] and during neurosurgery on patients with intracranial masses.[167,168] One of the most widely cited papers involved ten patients with intracranial masses given 1.5

mg/kg of lidocaine or placebo at the time of induction after receiving diazepam, atropine, and morphine one hour prior to intubation. The group with placebo (saline) pretreatment had a 12 mmHg ICP increase for one minute during intubation that resolved with general anesthesia while the lidocaine group's ICP did not measurably increase ($p < 0.05$).[167]

Like the prior study, 20 patients with intracranial pressure monitors undergoing anesthesia with morphine, diazepam and atropine pre-treatment received either lidocaine or thiopental in response to elevated intracranial pressure elevations. Both groups showed similar small reductions in ICP. However, this study lacked a control group and received multiple agents that contributed to analgesia and sedation.[168]

A ten-patient crossover randomized controlled trial (RCT) involving patients intubated in the ICU with head injuries evaluated the effect of intravenous lidocaine on suctioning. All patients concurrently received a combination of steroids, mannitol and barbiturates. Two minutes prior to endotracheal suctioning, lidocaine was administered. In both groups (placebo and lidocaine), ICP increased by 10-12 mmHg with no statistical significance between groups. An unblinded RCT involving thiopental vs lidocaine prior to suctioning found no effect on ICP or mean arterial pressure during suctioning.[169]

No studies were directly performed on patients in the emergency department and all the studies to date use a mix of sedatives and analgesics that make definitive interpretation of lidocaine's effect difficult. Also, the suction and intubation attempts and techniques in the publications are generally poorly described, and no patient-centered outcomes such as neurologic survival or mortality have been assessed with respect to lidocaine. Given the lack of demonstrated patient-centered benefit, it is worth acknowledging that lidocaine is not without adverse events. Lidocaine carries the potential harm of allergic reactions and induced high-grade heart blocks, especially if dosed incorrectly.[170]

Since lidocaine requires two to three minutes prior to intubation to blunt the cough reflex or transient ICP elevation, the addition of a medication without a demonstrated clinical benefit only adds potential for complications during a stressful resuscitation.[61] Most importantly, an appropriately dosed induction agent provides the best protection against transient catecholamine surges during laryngoscopy, potentially negating the need for lidocaine.[171–173]

The Bottom Line

- Multiple studies suggest that lidocaine administration can provide at best a transient and mild blunting of ICP rise during laryngeal manipulation or suctioning.

- Lidocaine administration prior to suctioning is unlikely to blunt transient ICP increases.

- No patient-centered benefits have been demonstrated.

- Adequately dosed induction agents provide the best protection against transient catecholamine surges during laryngoscopy.

Morbidly obese patients can have CT or MRI imaging performed at the zoo

Daniel G. Ostermayer

The origin

When patients exceed the weight or width limits of emergency department computed tomography (CT) and magnetic resonance imaging (MRI) scanners, providers and staff frequently suggest the local zoo as an option for advanced imaging with heavier weight limits.[174,175] Of nationally surveyed zoos, 62% report being contacted by local hospitals with the request for advanced imaging of obese patients.[176]

The Facts

Unfortunately, the option to use zoo and veterinary hospital imaging modalities has no factual basis. Not only do most zoos not have advanced imaging, even if it were available, there is an unwillingness to image humans. In a telephone survey of 145 zoos and 28 veterinary hospitals, two zoos (1%) had CT scanners and neither would image human patients. Among veterinary schools, 16 (57%) had large weight capacity CT equipment, but only 4 (14%) would consider imaging human patients.[177] Another similar survey of nationally registered zoos confirmed the findings that most zoos do not have CT scanners and even if available would not image humans.[176] A zoo, even if available with scanning capacity, would face potential medicolegal liability, reimbursement difficulty (zoos do not contract with human insurance companies), and concerns with technician education (veterinary vs human imaging certifications). The only viable option for hospitals with morbidly obese patients is transfer to a hospital with bariatric imaging capabilities.[178]

The Bottom Line

- Most zoos lack advanced imaging available for morbidly obese adults.

- Zoos and veterinary hospitals that have imaging capabilities will not image humans.

Patients with NSTEMIs should receive heparin

Daniel G. Ostermayer

The origin

The use of heparin for noninvasive management of a non-ST-elevation myocardial infarction (NSTEMI) stems from misunderstandings of historic science. Physiologically, heparin prevents thrombosis by extending clotting times and can also reduce propagation of an existing thrombus. Patients with NSTEMIs who have acute thrombotic coronary occlusions, in theory, would benefit from heparinization.[179] The 2014 American Heart Association guidelines for the management of NSTEMI recommend unfractionated heparin with an initial loading dose of 60 IU/kg (maximum 4,000 IU) followed by an infusion of 12 IU/kg/hr (maximum 1,000 IU/hr) for patients undergoing percutaneous coronary intervention (PCI).[180]

The Facts

The use of empiric anticoagulation for patients with unstable angina or NSTEMIs originated from the early PCI literature. During PCI, interventional wire and ballooning can cause vascular trauma and arterial irritation which can promote thrombosis.[181] The empiric anticoagulation helps prevent these procedural complications and improves outcomes.[182] Although heparin remains the most commonly used systemic anticoagulant to reduce thrombosis during PCI, other anticoagulants such as bivalirudin have been used.[183] Systemic anticoagulation during PCI is not used to treat the acute coronary thrombosis, but rather to reduce the periprocedural thrombotic complications.[184–186]

A series of randomized trials have attempted to establish a patient-centered benefit to empiric heparinization for patients with an NSTEMI outside of those receiving anticoagulation for the PCI. The first randomized controlled trial (RCT) in 1988 included 479 patients with unstable angina receiving PCI who were randomized to placebo, aspirin, heparin infusion, or both. Although all patients demonstrated a reduction in infarction and refractory angina, there was no statistical difference with regard to any endpoint (refractory angina, myocardial infarction, or death).[187]

Subsequent studies comparing aspirin to aspirin plus heparin in unstable angina have also failed to find a morbidity or mortality benefit.[188–191] When combining the RCTs in a meta-analysis, the results approached but did not achieve statistical significance in reducing myocardial infarction or death (risk ratio 0.67; 95% CI 0.44-1.02). When extending the timeframe beyond hospitalization to include 2 to 12 weeks after randomization, the confidence intervals were even wider (risk ratio 0.82; 95% CI 0.56-1.20).

The most important trials, FRISC[191] and RISC,[188] showed that heparin caused an initial reduction in myocardial infarction but was associated with a rebound in infarction after cessation of heparinization. These randomized trials used patients with unstable angina, which would most likely be diagnosed with NSTEMI in the current era of high and ultra-high sensitivity troponin assays.

While awaiting a planned PCI, there may be a benefit for anticoagulation if it outweighs any possible bleeding risks (3-4% increase in risk).[192] If PCI is not planned, the current evidence does not support heparinization. Prior to a planned PCI, heparinization could be started within a short period of time rather than maintaining a prolonged infusion.

The Facts

- Empiric heparinization for patients with an NSTEMI does not reduce long-term morbidity or mortality.

- Heparin as a therapy for patients with unstable angina and NSTEMI originated from the PCI literature as a means of reducing procedural complications.

- Despite guideline recommendations, heparin has no supporting evidence in patients with NSTEMI not undergoing PCI.

Combine lidocaine with bupivacaine for nerve blocks to achieve fast and long acting analgesia

Daniel G. Ostermayer

The Origin

Combining lidocaine (1-2%) and bupivacaine (0.25-5%) for nerve blocks stems from the misunderstanding that bupivacaine has a longer onset of action than lidocaine. Providers will often create a one-to-one mixture of lidocaine and bupivacaine with the goal of achieving a fast onset nerve block (from lidocaine) with a long duration of action (from bupivacaine).[193]

The Facts

In ideal conditions, bupivacaine (0.5%) provides an average of 25 hours of anesthesia compared to ten hours from 2% lidocaine with epinephrine (1:100,000), and five hours from 2% lidocaine without epinephrine.[194] Lidocaine has time to onset of 1-3 minutes and bupivacaine of 2-10 minutes.[193] Two randomized controlled trials (RCTs) have assessed the differences between lidocaine, bupivacaine and one-to-one mixtures for regional anesthesia.

The first study was a double-blind experiment that included twelve medical student volunteers in which both deep peroneal nerves were anesthetized using one of the three options: (1) 1% lidocaine, (2) 0.25% bupivacaine, or

(3) a one-to-one mixture of both. The other side was injected with saline as a control. Although likely underpowered, the study failed to demonstrate a statistical difference for the time of onset (mean 80-100 sec, p = 0.63) of anesthesia using a monofilament sensation test between groups. As expected, the mean duration of bupivacaine alone was nine hours; significantly longer than lidocaine or one-to-one mixture group (3.5 hours).[193]

The second RCT performed digital blocks in healthy volunteers who were randomized to lidocaine (1%) with epinephrine or bupivacaine (0.5%). The median time to anesthesia was not significantly different between the two groups (3.4 minutes vs 3.3 minutes, p = 0.84). The median time needed for return of pinprick sensation was significantly different between the two drugs (321 minutes for lidocaine vs 701 minutes for bupivacaine, p < 0.05). The bupivacaine group, however, experienced greater initial pain during injection than the lidocaine with epinephrine group.

Bupivacaine, in clinical practice, provides a similar onset of action to lidocaine or a one-to-one mixture, but bupivacaine alone has a significantly longer duration of action. Although pain reduction may be accomplished by mixing anesthetics (reducing the amount of bupivacaine), the desired duration of action is significantly less. Buffering either anesthetic with sodium bicarbonate may decrease the pain of injection.[194]

Clinicians should choose their anesthetic based on the duration of action and not the time of onset since both bupivacaine and lidocaine provide similar times to initial anesthesia. A mixture of bupivacaine and lidocaine only increase procedural complexity and shortens the absolute duration of analgesia.

The Bottom Line

- Lidocaine and bupivacaine both provide an onset of action within approximately three minutes.

- Mixing anesthetics only decreases the duration of analgesia.

- Buffering the anesthetic with sodium bicarbonate may reduce the pain associated with lidocaine or bupivacaine injections.

Against Medical Advice designations should be used for patients leaving before treatment completion

Manpreet Singh, Daniel G. Ostermayer

The Origin

Against medical advice (AMA) discharges account for 1-2% of all discharges in the United States[195] and the United Kingdom.[196] Patients of lower socioeconomic classes and those in economically disadvantaged urban areas compose a greater proportion of AMA discharges.[197,198] Emergency departments and hospitals widely employ AMA forms or AMA designations for patients leaving prior to treatment or evaluation completion. Most providers also assume that signing an AMA form offers a degree of medicolegal protection, since these patients generally carry a greater risk of morbidity and mortality as well as greater rates of readmissions.[195,197,198]

The Facts

A medical malpractice negligence case against a provider requires establishment of a direct line of evidence that the provider had a duty to the patient that was breached and directly led to the patient's harm.[199] An AMA form, although intended as documentation that the provider no longer has a duty to treat the patient due to the patient's refusal of care, offers little to no legal protection. In fact, the AMA designation itself offers no legal protection and has no legal mandate.

Although case law has established that a patient ends the doctor-patient relationship when leaving AMA,[200,201] the only means of protection for the physician stems from the appropriateness and safety of an AMA discharge regardless of the patient signing a form.[202] Since the process of establishing a safe AMA is the same process employed when establishing a safe discharge, the AMA process only works to create an adversarial doctor-patient encounter.[203] Compared to patients discharged conventionally from an emergency department, 25% of patients discharged AMA reported not wanting to return for follow-up care.[204,205]

Multiple U.S. legal cases address termination of the physician-patient relationship in cases where patients left a hospital without informing their primary physician or cases where a physician described risks of harm and potential benefits, yet the patient left prior to treatment completion. In all cases where the physician was found to no longer have a duty to the patient, it was after the patient was given all necessary information and had decisional capacity yet still left care.[200] The designation in the medical chart (AMA vs discharge) had no bearing on the legal rulings. The process of discussing risks and benefits, treatment options, and establishing decisional capacity are the exact processes that must take place during a normal discharge. This makes the AMA designation irrelevant.

Patients leaving AMA must have capacity to refuse care, should receive an explanation of all potential risks of leaving and potential benefits to staying, and this process should be documented in the chart.[200] If these conditions are not met and not documented, the AMA process can be questioned and the physician's duty may have been breached, placing them at legal risk. Although an AMA discharge form is thought to be a formal way to distance oneself from an unsafe discharge, if decisional capacity and explanation of harms and benefits is absent from documentation, the form has no legal or clinical value.[206]

Hospitals may have a financial incentive to encourage physicians to utilize AMA forms. Medicare's Hospital Readmission Reduction Program excludes initial admissions ending in an AMA discharge from 30-day readmission penalties. Since patients leaving prior to completion of their care are at greater risk, hospital systems seek to buffer themselves against the potential readmission penalty. However, readmission reduction has no bearing on patients receiving emergency department workups who have not been admitted.[207]

The Bottom Line

- AMA forms provide no value in the emergency department and most likely should not be used.

- The process of patient discharge, not the AMA form or AMA designation, offers legal protection to clinicians.

- Patients leaving prior to treatment completion should have documented competency and receive an appropriate explanation enabling understanding of risks and benefits.

- The AMA designation creates a potentially adversarial environment and only benefits hospitals seeking to avoid readmission penalties for inpatients.

Etomidate induction causes adrenal suppression and should be avoided in critically ill patients

Miles R. Maassen, Daniel G. Ostermayer

The Origin

Physicians first used etomidate for anesthetic induction in Europe in 1972.[208] It showed promise as an alternative to thiopental and barbiturates for anesthetic induction, since the drug caused no histamine release and would not worsen bronchospasm in critical asthmatics. Etomidate also did not suppress cardiac function and maintained hemodynamic stability. Initially the only reported adverse effect was transient myoclonic jerks.[209]

Beginning in the 1980s, etomidate gained increasing use as an infusion for sedation in intensive care units (ICUs). In 1983, *The Lancet* published a report on the association between etomidate and increased mortality of critically ill trauma patients in the United Kingdom. The retrospective review of records from 1979 to 1982 described how benzodiazepines served as the standard sedative prior to etomidate infusions. Although injury severity scores remained constant over the time period, mortality increased from 25% to 44% with etomidate being the only notable change in the ICUs studied. The authors suggested etomidate's effect on steroid production as a cause of increased mortality, since the

69

drug affected patients' responsiveness to adrenocorticotropic hormone stimulation tests.[210]

In 1984, in vitro studies confirmed etomidate's effect on cortisol production by inhibiting 11-beta-hydroxylase.[211] Concerns of adrenal suppression increased further after publication of a case series of gynecologic patients undergoing laparotomy. Patients received either thiopental or etomidate inductions (0.35 mg/kg). Cortisol levels measured during surgery decreased below pre-operative measurements in both the thiopental and etomidate induction groups. The etomidate group, however, required as long as four hours to recover from the transient adrenal suppression.[212]

The Facts

In the 1990s and 2000s, initial concerns of adrenal suppression from etomidate infusions in ICUs, combined with concerns of steroid responsiveness in septic patients, led to skepticism over etomidate's use in critical patients.[213] It stands to reason that if patients had relative adrenal suppression as a result of septic shock, any medication (like etomidate) that causes transient adrenal suppression should be avoided. However, there has never been a reliable association demonstrated between a single induction dose of etomidate and mortality. In the first randomized controlled trial (RCT) of its kind, 35 critical patients were randomized to a single induction dose of thiopental or etomidate. Although cortisol response from an adrenocorticotropic-hormone-stimulation test was blunted in the etomidate group, no mortality difference was observed in this small sample.[214]

Two major studies provided further evidence against an association of etomidate with increased mortality. Annane et al. randomized patients with septic shock and relative adrenal insufficiency to receive either hydrocortisone and fludrocortisone or placebo.[215] As expected, etomidate blunted response to adrenocorticotropic hormone stimulation, but patients with adrenal non-response had the same mortality as those with etomidate-associated non-response (53% vs 54.8%).[216] The retrospective CORTICUS study (which established baseline cortisol and adrenocorticotropic-hormone -stimulation response in sepsis) also confirmed that etomidate suppresses adrenal response to adrenocorticotropic hormone stimulation. After adjusting for severity of sepsis, no association between etomidate and mortality was found (OR, 1.82; 95% CI, 0.52-6.36).[217]

Two non-interventional studies of septic shock patients admitted to the ICU also failed to find an association with the induction agent and clinical outcomes.[218,219] The only emergency-department study randomized consecutive patients requiring intubation to midazolam or etomidate followed by succinylcholine. Although response to corticotropin stimulation was depressed in the etomidate group for up to 12 hours, cortisol levels remained within normal limits through the period of dysfunction.[220]

Trauma patients also experience a similar decline in their cortisol production and response to adrenocorticotropic hormone stimulation when given induction dose etomidate.[221] However, no mortality difference was found between ketamine and etomidate.[222] Trauma patients admitted to the Royal London Hospital trauma ICU who received varying weight-based doses of etomidate for induction did not demonstrate adrenal suppression after 18 hours.[223] For septic pediatric patients, a retrospective study of 60 children confirmed results consistent with the adult literature. Etomidate blunts response to adrenocorticotropic hormone stimulation. A study of children with meningitis by den Brinker et al. reported eight deaths, with seven of those patients having received induction dose etomidate; however, this was a retrospective study at risk of bias with a small sample size. Of note, in this study, 23 of the 31 intubated children received etomidate induction.[224] Although etomidate blunts adrenal stimulation response, the speed of induction and hemodynamic neutrality may reduce the harms of hypotension that can occur during the intubation of the critically ill.[225,226]

The Bottom Line

* Etomidate suppresses adrenal response to adrenocorticotropic hormone stimulation by inhibiting 11-beta-hydroxylase.

* A single induction dose of etomidate for has not been shown to impact mortality.

* Etomidate infusions may lead to prolonged adrenal suppression and increase mortality.

* The hemodynamic neutrality of etomidate allows for safe intubating conditions for critically ill patients.

References

1.   Barkun A, Sabbah S, Enns R, et al. The Canadian Registry on Nonvariceal Upper Gastrointestinal Bleeding and Endoscopy (RUGBE): Endoscopic hemostasis and proton pump inhibition are associated with improved outcomes in a real-life setting. *Am J Gastroenterol.* 2004;99(7):1238-1246.

2.   Silverstein FE, Gilbert DA, Tedesco FJ, Buenger NK, Persing J. The national ASGE survey on upper gastrointestinal bleeding. II. Clinical prognostic factors. *Gastrointest Endosc.* 1981;27(2):80-93.

3.   Kolkman JJ, Meuwissen SG. A review on treatment of bleeding peptic ulcer: a collaborative task of gastroenterologist and surgeon. *Scand J Gastroenterol Suppl.* 1996;218(sup218):16-25.

4.   Chaimoff C, Creter D, Djaldetti M. The effect of pH on platelet and coagulation factor activities. *Am J Surg.* 1978;136(2):257-259.

5.   Green FW, Kaplan MM, Curtis LE, Levine PH. Effect of acid and pepsin on blood coagulation and platelet aggregation. A possible contributor prolonged gastroduodenal mucosal hemorrhage. *Gastroenterology.* 1978;74(1):38-43.

6.   Gralnek IM, Barkun AN, Bardou M. Management of acute bleeding from a peptic ulcer. *N Engl J Med.*

2008;359(9):928-937.

7.   Huggins RM, Scates AC, Latour JK. Intravenous proton-pump inhibitors versus H2-antagonists for treatment of GI bleeding. *Ann Pharmacother.* 2003;37(3):433-437.

8.   Ali Khan M, Howden CW. The Role of Proton Pump Inhibitors in the Management of Upper Gastrointestinal Disorders. *Gastroenterol Hepatol (N Y).* 2018;14(3):169-175.

9.   Levine JE, Leontiadis GI, Sharma VK, Howden CW. Meta-analysis: the efficacy of intravenous H2-receptor antagonists in bleeding peptic ulcer. *Aliment Pharmacol Ther.* 2002;16(6):1137-1142.

10. Kiilerich S, Rannem T, Elsborg L. Effect of intravenous infusion of omeprazole and ranitidine on twenty-four-hour intragastric pH in patients with a history of duodenal ulcer. *Digestion.* 1995;56(1):25-30.

11. Netzer P, Gaia C, Sandoz M, et al. Effect of repeated injection and continuous infusion of omeprazole and ranitidine on intragastric pH over 72 hours. *Am J Gastroenterol.* 1999;94(2):351-357.

12. Wang K, Lin H-J, Perng C-L, et al. The effect of H2-receptor antagonist and proton pump inhibitor on microbial proliferation in the stomach. *Hepatogastroenterology.* 51(59):1540-1543.

13. Barkun AN, Cockeram AW, Plourde V, Fedorak RN. Acid suppression in non-variceal acute upper gastrointestinal bleeding. *Aliment Pharmacol Ther.* 1999;13(12):1565-1584.

14. Sreedharan A, Martin J, Leontiadis GI, et al. Proton pump inhibitor treatment initiated prior to endoscopic diagnosis in upper gastrointestinal bleeding. *Cochrane database Syst Rev.* 2010; (7):CD005415.

15. Daneshmend TK, Hawkey CJ, Langman MJS, Logan RFA, Long RG, Walt RP. Omeprazole versus placebo for acute upper gastrointestinal bleeding: randomised double blind controlled trial. *BMJ.* 1992;304(6820):143-147.

16. Lau JYW, Sung JJY, Lee KK, et al. Effect of intravenous omeprazole on recurrent bleeding after endoscopic treatment of bleeding peptic ulcers. *N Engl J Med.* 2000;343(5):310-316.

17. Lau JY, Leung WK, Wu JCY, et al. Omeprazole before endoscopy in patients with gastrointestinal bleeding. *N Engl J Med.* 2007;356(16):1631-1640.

18. Gralnek IM, Dumonceau JM, Kuipers EJ, et al. Diagnosis and management of nonvariceal upper gastrointestinal hemorrhage: European Society of Gastrointestinal Endoscopy (ESGE) Guideline. *Endoscopy.* 2015;47(10):a1-a46.

19.   NICE. Acute upper gastrointestinal bleeding in over 16s : management. *Natl Inst Heal Care Excell.* 2012;(June):1-23.

20.   Sung JJY, Chiu PWY, Chan FKL, et al. Asia-Pacific working group consensus on non-variceal upper gastrointestinal bleeding: An update 2018. *Gut.* 2018;67(10):1757-1768.

21.   Sung JJY, Chan FKL, Lau JYW, et al. The Effect of Endoscopic Therapy in Patients Receiving Omeprazole for Bleeding Ulcers with Nonbleeding Visible Vessels or Adherent Clots. *Ann Intern Med.* 2003;139(4):237.

22.   Laine L, McQuaid KR. Endoscopic Therapy for Bleeding Ulcers: An Evidence-Based Approach Based on Meta-Analyses of Randomized Controlled Trials. *Clin Gastroenterol Hepatol.* 2009;7(1):33-47.

23.   Leontiadis GI, Sreedharan A, Dorward S, et al. Systematic reviews of the clinical effectiveness and cost-effectiveness of proton pump inhibitors in acute upper gastrointestinal bleeding. *Health Technol Assess.* 2007;11(51):iii-iv, 1-164.

24.   Wilkes JJ. The Creation of HIPAA Culture: Prioritizing Privacy Paranoia over Patient Care. *Brigh Young Univ Law Rev.* 2014;2014(5):1213-1249.

25. Mullner R, Rafalski EM. Health Insurance Portability and Accountability Act of 1996 (HIPAA). *Encycl Heal Serv Res.* 2015.

26. De M. Understanding HIPAA, and how it can hurt health care. 2016:5-8.

27. Span P. Hipaa's Use as Code of Silence Often Misinterprets the Law. The New York Times.

28. Berwick DM, Gaines ME. How HIPAA harms care, and how to stop it. *JAMA - J Am Med Assoc.* 2018;320(3):229-230.

29. Macrobert RG. The cause of lumbar puncture headache. *J Am Med Assoc.* 1918;70(19):1350-1353.

30. Calverley RK, Scheller M. Anesthesia as a specialty: past, present, and future. *Clin Anesth.* 1989;17:947.

31. Kunkle EC, Ray BS, Wolff HG. Experimental studies on headache: analysis of the headache associated with changes in intracranial pressure. *Arch Neurol Psychiatry.* 1943;49(3):323-358.

32. Nelson MO. Postpuncture headaches: A clinical and experimental study of the cause and prevention. *Arch Derm Syphilol.* 1930;21(4):615-627.

33. Alpers BJ. LUMBAR PUNCTURE HEADACHE. *Arch Neurol Psychiatry.* 1925;14(6):806.

34. Dana CL. Puncture headache. *J Am Med Assoc.* 1917;LXVIII(14):1017.

35. Torbert HC. THE SAFETY OF LUMBAR PUNCTURE FOR AMBULATORY PATIENTS. *Arch Dermatol.* 1934;30(5):692.

36. Carbaat PA, van Crevel H. Lumbar puncture headache: controlled study on the preventive effect of 24 hours' bed rest. *Lancet (London, England).* 1981;2(8256):1133-1135.

37. Arevalo-Rodriguez I, Ciapponi A, Roqué i Figuls M, Muñoz L, Bonfill Cosp X. Posture and fluids for preventing post-dural puncture headache. *Cochrane database Syst Rev.* 2016;3(3):CD009199.

38. Turnbull DK, Shepherd DB. Post-dural puncture headache: pathogenesis, prevention and treatment. *Br J Anaesth.* 2003;91(5):718-729.

39. Arevalo-Rodriguez I, Muñoz L, Godoy-Casasbuenas N, et al. Needle gauge and tip designs for preventing post-dural puncture headache (PDPH). *Cochrane Database Syst Rev.* 2017;42(10):1209-1214.

40. Flaatten H, Thorsen T, Askeland B, et al. Puncture technique and postural postdural puncture headache. A randomised, double-blind study comparing transverse and parallel puncture. *Acta*

Anaesthesiol Scand. 1998;42(10):1209-1214.

41. Strupp M, Brandt T, Müller A. Incidence of post-lumbar puncture syndrome reduced by reinserting the stylet: A randomized prospective study of 600 patients. *J Neurol.* 1998;245(9):589-592.

42. Jarvis AP, Greenawalt JW, Fagraeus L. Intravenous caffeine for postdural puncture headache. *Anesth Analg.* 1986;65(3):316-317.

43. Yücel A, Ozyalçin S, Talu GK, Yücel EC, Erdine S. Intravenous administration of caffeine sodium benzoate for postdural puncture headache. *Reg Anesth Pain Med.* 1999;24(1):51-54.

44. RAINBIRD A, PFITZNER J. Restricted spread of analgesia following epidural blood patch. Case report with a review of possible complications. *Anaesthesia.* 1983;38(5):481-484.

45. Ahmed S V., Jayawarna C, Jude E. Post lumbar puncture headache: Diagnosis and management. *Postgrad Med J.* 2006;82(973):713-716.

46. Kovalak M, Lake J, Mattek N, Eisen G, Lieberman D, Zaman A. Endoscopic screening for varices in cirrhotic patients: data from a national endoscopic database. *Gastrointest Endosc.* 2007;65(1):82-88.

47. Sen S, Williams R, Jalan R. The pathophysiological basis of acute-on-chronic liver failure. *Liver.* 2002;22(SUPPL. 2):5-13.

48. Hon WM, Lee KH, Khoo HE. Nitric oxide in liver diseases: friend, foe, or just passerby? *Ann N Y Acad Sci*. 2002;962(65):275-295.

49. Hanisch E, Doertenbach J, Usadel KH. Somatostatin in acute bleeding oesophageal varices. Pharmacology and rationale for use. *Drugs*. 1992;44 Suppl 2(2):24-35; discussion 70-2.

50. LaBrecque D, Khan AG, Sarin SK, Le Mair AW. World Gastroenterology Organisation Global Guidelines, esophageal varices. *Milwaukee, Wisconsin World Gastroenterol Organ*. 2014:2-11.

51. Jalan R, Hayes PC. UK guidelines on the management of variceal haemorrhage in cirrhotic patients. British Society of Gastroenterology. *Gut*. 2000;46 Suppl 3(11):III1-III15.

52. Garcia-Tsao G, Sanyal AJ, Grace ND, Carey WD. Varices and variceal hemorrhage in cirrhosis. *Am J Gastroenterol*. 2007;102(9):2086-2102.

53. Besson I, Ingrand P, Person B, et al. Sclerotherapy with or without octreotide for acute variceal bleeding. *N Engl J Med*. 1995;333(9):555-560.

54. Gøtzsche PC, Hróbjartsson A. Somatostatin analogues for acute bleeding oesophageal varices. *Cochrane Database Syst Rev*. 2008;(3).

55. Bañares R, Albillos A, Rincón D, et al. Endoscopic treatment versus endoscopic plus pharmacologic

treatment for acute variceal bleeding: a meta-analysis. *Hepatology*. 2002;35(3):609-615.

56.   Corley DA, Cello JP, Adkisson W, Ko WF, Kerlikowske K. Octreotide for acute esophageal variceal bleeding: a meta-analysis. *Gastroenterology*. 2001;120(4):946-954.

57.   D'Amico G. First meta-analysis of octreotide for variceal bleeding. A lost opportunity. *J Hepatol*. 2002;36(4):574-577.

58.   Rubin AI, Howett GL. *Emergency Vehicle Warning Lights: State of the Art*. U.S. Department of Commerce National Bureau of Standards; 1978.

59.   Kuehl AE, Bill WH, Ryan L, It DRS. Use of warning lights and siren in emergency medical vehicle response and patient transport. National Association of Emergency Medical Services Physicians (NAEMSP) and the National Association of State EMS Directors (NASEMSD). *Prehosp Disaster Med*. 1994;9(2):133-136.

60.   Custalow CB, Gravitz CS. Emergency medical vehicle collisions and potential for preventive intervention. *Prehosp Emerg Care*. 2004;8(2):175-184.

61.   Clawson JJ, Martin RL, Cady GA, Maio RF. The Wake-Effect—Emergency Vehicle-Related Collisions. *Prehosp Disaster Med*.

1997;12(4):41-44.

62. Clawson JJ, Martin RL, Cady GA, Maio RF. The Wake-Effect—Emergency Vehicle-Related Collisions. *Prehosp Disaster Med.* 1997;12(4):41-44.

63. Kupas DF, Dula DJ, Pino BJ. Patient outcome using medical protocol to limit "lights and siren" transport. *Prehosp Disaster Med.* 1994;9(4):226-229.

64. Clawson JJ. Running "hot" and the case of Sharron Rose. *JEMS.* 1991;16(7):11-13.

65. Ho J, Casey B. Time saved with use of emergency warning lights and sirens during response to requests for emergency medical aid in an urban environment. *Ann Emerg Med.* 1998;32(5):585-588.

66. Brown LH, Whitney CL, Hunt RC, Addario M, Hogue T. Do warning lights and sirens reduce ambulance response times? *Prehosp Emerg Care.* 1999;4(1):70-74.

67. Rawles JM, Kenmure AC. Controlled trial of oxygen in uncomplicated myocardial infarction. *Br Med J.* 1976;1(6018):1121-1123.

68. Stub D, Smith K, Bernard S, et al. Air Versus Oxygen in ST-Segment-Elevation Myocardial Infarction. *Circulation.* 2015;131(24):2143-2150.

69. Cabello JB, Burls A, Emparanza JI, Bayliss SE, Quinn T. Oxygen therapy for acute myocardial infarction. *Cochrane database Syst Rev.* 2016;12(12):CD007160.

70. Hofmann R, James SK, Jernberg T, et al. Oxygen Therapy in Suspected Acute Myocardial Infarction. *N Engl J Med.* 2017;377(13):1240-1249.

71. Sepehrvand N, James SK, Stub D, Khoshnood A, Ezekowitz JA, Hofmann R. Effects of supplemental oxygen therapy in patients with suspected acute myocardial infarction: a meta-analysis of randomised clinical trials. *Heart.* 2018;104(20):1691-1698.

72. Dundee JW, Loan WB, Morrison JD. Studies of drugs given before anaesthesia. XIX. The opiates. *Br J Anaesth.* 1970;42(1):54-58.

73. Roberts GW, Bekker TB, Carlsen HH, et al. Postoperative nausea and vomiting are strongly influenced by postoperative opioid use in a dose-related manner. *Anesth Analg.* 2005;101(5):1343-1348.

74. Chung F, Lane R, Spraggs C, et al. Ondansetron is more effective than metoclopramide for the treatment of opioid-induced emesis in post-surgical adult patients. Ondansetron OIE Post-Surgical Study Group. *Eur J Anaesthesiol.*

1999;16(10):669-677.

75. Smith HS, Laufer A. Opioid induced nausea and vomiting. *Eur J Pharmacol.* 2014;722(1):67-78.

76. Lambie B, Chambers J, Herbison P. The role of prophylatic anti-emetic therapy in emergency department patients receiving intravenous morphine for musculoskeletal trauma. *Emerg Med.* 1999;11(4):240-243.

77. Talbot-Stern J, Paoloni R. Prophylactic metoclopramide is unnecessary with intravenous analgesia in the ED. *Am J Emerg Med.* 2000;18(6):653-657.

78. Bradshaw M, Sen A. Use of a prophylactic antiemetic with morphine in acute pain: Randomised controlled trial. *Emerg Med J.* 2006;23(3):210-213.

79. Hafermann MJ, Namdar R, Seibold GE, Page RL. Effect of intravenous ondansetron on QT interval prolongation in patients with cardiovascular disease and additional risk factors for torsades: a prospective, observational study. *Drug Healthc Patient Saf.* 2011;3(4):53-58.

80. Culver MA, Richards EC, Jarrell DH, Edwards CJ. Use of Prophylactic Ondansetron with Intravenous Opioids in Emergency Department Patients: A Prospective Observational Pilot Study. *J Emerg*

Med. 2017;53(5):629-634.

81. McKimm-Breschkin JL. Influenza neuraminidase inhibitors: antiviral action and mechanisms of resistance. *Influenza Other Respi Viruses.* 2013;7 Suppl 1(1 SUPPL.1):25-36.

82. Payne D. Tamiflu: the battle for secret drug data. *BMJ.* 2012;345(7881):e7303.

83. Treanor JJ, Hayden FG, Vrooman PS, et al. Efficacy and Safety of the Oral Neuraminidase Inhibitor Oseltamivir in Treating Acute Influenza. *JAMA.* 2000;283(8):1016.

84. Nicholson K, Aoki F, Osterhaus A, et al. Efficacy and safety of oseltamivir in treatment of acute influenza: a randomised controlled trial. *Lancet.* 2000;355(9218):1845-1850.

85. Hsu J, Santesso N, Mustafa R, et al. Antivirals for Treatment of Influenza. *Ann Intern Med.* 2012;156(7):512.

86. Kaiser L, Wat C, Mills T, Mahoney P, Ward P, Hayden F. Impact of oseltamivir treatment on influenza-related lower respiratory tract complications and hospitalizations. *Arch Intern Med.* 2003;163(14):1667-1672.

87. Po ALW, Farndon P, Palmer N. Maximizing the value of drug stockpiles for pandemic influenza. *Emerg Infect Dis.* 2009;15(10):1686-1687.

88. Vilhelmsson A, Mulinari S. Pharmaceutical lobbying and pandemic stockpiling of Tamiflu: A qualitative study of arguments and tactics. *J Public Heal (United Kingdom)*. 2018;40(3):646-651.

89. Jefferson T, Jones MA, Doshi P, et al. Neuraminidase inhibitors for preventing and treating influenza in healthy adults and children. *Cochrane database Syst Rev*. 2014;(4):CD008965.

90. Dobson J, Whitley RJ, Pocock S, Monto AS. Oseltamivir treatment for influenza in adults: a meta-analysis of randomised controlled trials. *Lancet (London, England)*. 2015;385(9979):1729-1737.

91. Nakamura Y, Sugawara T, Ohkusa Y, et al. Life-threatening abnormal behavior incidence in 10-19 year old patients administered neuraminidase inhibitors. *PLoS One*. 2015;10(7):1-8.

92. Kitching A, Roche A, Balasegaram S, Heathcock R, Maguire H. Oseltamivir adherence and side effects among children in three London schools affected by influenza A(H1N1)v, May 2009 - an internet-based cross-sectional survey. *Euro Surveill*. 2009;14(30):19287.

93. Toovey S, Prinssen EP, Rayner CR, et al. Post-marketing assessment of neuropsychiatric adverse events in influenza patients treated with

oseltamivir: An updated review. *Adv Ther.* 2012;29(10):826-848.

94. Cohen D. Complications: tracking down the data on oseltamivir. *BMJ.* 2009;339:b5387.

95. Dunn AG, Arachi D, Hudgins J, Tsafnat G, Coiera E, Bourgeois FT. Financial conflicts of interest and conclusions about neuraminidase inhibitors for influenza: an analysis of systematic reviews. *Ann Intern Med.* 2014;161(7):513-518.

96. Butler CC, van der Velden AW, Bongard E, et al. Oseltamivir plus usual care versus usual care for influenza-like illness in primary care: an open-label, pragmatic, randomised controlled trial. *Lancet.* 2020;395(10217):42-52.

97. Laursen SB, Jørgensen HS, Schaffalitzky de Muckadell OB. National consensus on management of peptic ulcer bleeding in Denmark 2014. *Dan Med J.* 2014;61(11):1-10.

98. Perng CL, Lin HJ, Chen CJ, Lee FY, Lee SD, Lee CH. Characteristics of patients with bleeding peptic ulcer requiring emergency endoscopy and aggressive treatment. *Am J Gastroenterol.* 1994;89(10):1811-1814.

99. Srygley FD, Gerardo CJ, Tran T, Fisher DA. Does this patient have a severe upper gastrointestinal bleed? *JAMA - J Am Med Assoc.*

2012;307(10):1072-1079.

100. Palamidessi N, Sinert R, Falzon L, Zehtabchi S. Nasogastric aspiration and lavage in emergency department patients with hematochezia or melena without hematemesis. *Acad Emerg Med.* 2010;17(2):126-132.

101. Singer AJ, Richman PB, Kowalska A, Thode J. Comparison of patient and practitioner assessments of pain from commonly performed emergency department procedures. *Ann Emerg Med.* 1999;33(6):652-658.

102. Aljebreen AM, Fallone CA, Barkun AN. Nasogastric aspirate predicts high-risk endoscopic lesions in patients with acute upper-GI bleeding. *Gastrointest Endosc.* 2004;59(2):172-178.

103. Cappell MS. Safety and efficacy of nasogastric intubation for gastrointestinal bleeding after myocardial infarction: An analysis of 125 patients at two tertiary cardiac referral hospitals. *Dig Dis Sci.* 2005;50(11):2063-2070.

104. Pateron D, Vicaut E, Debuc E, et al. Erythromycin infusion or gastric lavage for upper gastrointestinal bleeding: A multicenter randomized controlled trial. *Ann Emerg Med.* 2011;57(6):582-589.

105. Huang ES, Karsan S, Kanwal F, Singh I, Makhani M, Spiegel BM. Impact of nasogastric lavage on

outcomes in acute GI bleeding. *Gastrointest Endosc.* 2011;74(5):971-980.

106. Marder VJ, Francis CW. Plasmin degradation of cross-linked fibrin. *Ann N Y Acad Sci.* 1983;408(1):397-406.

107. GAFFNEY PJ, EDGELL T, CREIGHTON-KEMPSFORD LJ, WHEELER S, TARELLI E. Fibrin degradation product (FnDP) assays: analysis of standardization issues and target antigens in plasma. *Br J Haematol.* 1995;90(1):187-194.

108. Brown MD, Rowe BH, Reeves MJ, Bermingham JM, Goldhaber SZ. The accuracy of the enzyme-linked immunosorbent assay D-dimer test in the diagnosis of pulmonary embolism: a meta-analysis. *Ann Emerg Med.* 2002;40(2):133-144.

109. Chunilal SD, Brill-Edwards PA, Stevens PB, et al. The sensitivity and specificity of a red blood cell agglutination D-dimer assay for venous thromboembolism when performed on venous blood. *Arch Intern Med.* 2002;162(2):217-220.

110. Schutgens REG, Haas FJLM, Gerritsen WBM, Van Der Horst F, Nieuwenhuis HK, Biesma DH. The usefulness of five D-dimer assays in the exclusion of deep venous thrombosis. *J Thromb Haemost.* 2003;1(5):976-981.

111. Sanchez LD, McGillicuddy DC, Volz KA, Fan SL,

Joyce N, Horowitz GL. Effect of two different FDA-approved D-dimer assays on resource utilization in the emergency department. *Acad Emerg Med.* 2011;18(3):317-321.

112. Douma RA, Le Gal G, Söhne M, et al. Potential of an age adjusted D-dimer cut-off value to improve the exclusion of pulmonary embolism in older patients: A retrospective analysis of three large cohorts. *BMJ.* 2010;340(7753):962.

113. Penaloza A, Roy PM, Kline J, et al. Performance of age-adjusted D-dimer cut-off to rule out pulmonary embolism. *J Thromb Haemost.* 2012;10(7):1291-1296.

114. van Es J, Mos I, Douma R, et al. The combination of four different clinical decision rules and an age-adjusted D-dimer cut-off increases the number of patients in whom acute pulmonary embolism can safely be excluded. *Thromb Haemost.* 2012;107(1):167-171.

115. Fesmire FM, Brown MD, Espinosa JA, et al. Critical issues in the evaluation and management of adult patients presenting to the emergency department with suspected pulmonary embolism. *Ann Emerg Med.* 2011;57(6):628-652.e75.

116. Raja AS, Greenberg JO, Qaseem A, Denberg TD, Fitterman N, Schuur JD. Evaluation of patients with

suspected acute pulmonary embolism: Best practice advice from the Clinical Guidelines Committee of the American College of Physicians. *Ann Intern Med.* 2015;163(9):701-711.

117. Stein PD, Hull RD, Patel KC, et al. D-dimer for the exclusion of acute venous thrombosis and pulmonary embolism: a systematic review. *Ann Intern Med.* 2004;140(8):589-602.

118. Di Nisio M, Squizzato A, Rutjes AWS, Büller HR, Zwinderman AH, Bossuyt PMM. Diagnostic accuracy of D-dimer test for exclusion of venous thromboembolism: A systematic review. *J Thromb Haemost.* 2007;5(2):296-304.

119. Harper PL, Theakston E, Ahmed J, Ockelford P. D-dimer concentration increases with age reducing the clinical value of the D-dimer assay in the elderly. *Intern Med J.* 2007;37(9):607-613.

120. Kline JA, Kabrhel C. Emergency evaluation for pulmonary embolism, part 2: Diagnostic approach. *J Emerg Med.* 2015;49(1):104-117.

121. Sharp AL, Vinson DR, Alamshaw F, Handler J, Gould MK. An Age-Adjusted D-dimer Threshold for Emergency Department Patients with Suspected Pulmonary Embolus: Accuracy and Clinical Implications. *Ann Emerg Med.* 2016;67(2):249-257.

122. Righini M, Van Es J, Den Exter PL, et al. Age-

adjusted D-dimer cutoff levels to rule out pulmonary
embolism: The ADJUST-PE study. *JAMA - J Am Med Assoc.* 2014;311(11):1117-1124.

123. Gupta A, Raja AS, Ip IK, Khorasani R. Assessing 2 D-dimer age-adjustment strategies to optimize computed tomographic use in ED evaluation of pulmonary embolism. *Am J Emerg Med.* 2014;32(12):1499-1502.

124. Woller SC, Stevens SM, Adams DM, et al. Assessment of the Safety and Efficiency of Using an Age-Adjusted D-dimer Threshold to Exclude Suspected Pulmonary Embolism. *Chest.* 2014;146(6):1444-1451.

125. Schouten HJ, Geersing GJ, Koek HL, et al. Diagnostic accuracy of conventional or age adjusted D-dimer cut-off values in older patients with suspected venous thromboembolism: Systematic review and meta-analysis. *BMJ.* 2013;346(7910):1-13.

126. Tseng W-C, Wu M-H, Chen H-C, Kao F-Y, Huang S-K. Ventricular Fibrillation in a General Population – A National Database Study –. *Circ J.* 2016;80(11):2310-2316.

127. Kabrhel C, Van Hylckama Vlieg A, Muzikanski A, et al. Multicenter Evaluation of the YEARS Criteria in Emergency Department Patients Evaluated for

Pulmonary Embolism. *Acad Emerg Med.*
2018;25(9):987-994.

128. JANEWAY TC. A CLINICAL STUDY OF
HYPERTENSIVE CARDIOVASCULAR DISEASE.
Arch Intern Med. 1913;XII(6):755.

129. Vincent M, Wang S. Headache Classification
Committee of the International Headache Society
(IHS) The International Classification of Headache
Disorders, 3rd edition. *Cephalalgia.*
2018;38(1):1-211.

130. Saccò M, Meschi M, Regolisti G, et al. The
relationship between blood pressure and pain. *J
Clin Hypertens (Greenwich).* 2013;15(8):600-605.

131. Weiss NS. Relation of high blood pressure to
headache, epistaxis, and selected other symptoms.
The United States Health Examination Survey of
Adults. *N Engl J Med.* 1972;287(13):631-633.

132. Weiss NS. Relation of high blood pressure to
headache, epistaxis, and selected other symptoms.
The United States Health Examination Survey of
Adults. *N Engl J Med.* 1972;287(13):631-633.

133. Schéle R, Ahlborg B, Ekbom K. Physical
characteristics and allergic history in young men
with migraine and other headaches. *Headache.*
1978;18(2):80-86.

134. Kottke TE, Tuomilehto J, Puska P, Salonen JT. The

relationship of symptoms and blood pressure in a population sample. *Int J Epidemiol.* 1979;8(4):355-359.

135. Paulin JM, Waal-Manning HJ, Simpson FO, Knight RG. The prevalence of headache in a small New Zealand town. *Headache.* 1985;25(3):147-151.

136. D'Alessandro R, Benassi G, Lenzi PL, et al. Epidemiology of headache in the Republic of San Marino. *J Neurol Neurosurg Psychiatry.* 1988;51(1):21-27.

137. Ghione S. Hypertension-Associated Hypalgesia. *Hypertension.* 1996;28(3):494-504.

138. Hobson E V., Craven I, Catrin Blank S. Posterior reversible encephalopathy syndrome: A truly treatable neurologic illness. *Perit Dial Int.* 2012;32(6):590-594.

139. Lilja M. Withdrawal Syndromes and the Cessation of Antihypertensive Therapy. *Arch Intern Med.* 1982;142(4):839.

140. Shulman ST, Bisno AL, Clegg HW, et al. Clinical practice guideline for the diagnosis and management of group a streptococcal pharyngitis: 2012 update by the infectious diseases society of America. *Clin Infect Dis.* 2012;55(10):86-102.

141. DENNY FW. PREVENTION OF RHEUMATIC FEVER. *J Am Med Assoc.* 1950;143(2):151.

142. Denny FW, Wannamaker LW, Brink WR, Rammelkamp CH, Custer EA. Prevention of Rheumatic Fever: Treatment of the Preceding Streptococcic Infection. *JAMA J Am Med Assoc.* 1985;254(4):534-537.

143. Bisno AL. Group A Streptococcal Infections and Acute Rheumatic Fever. *N Engl J Med.* 1991;325(11):783-793.

144. Spinks A, Glasziou PP, Del Mar CB. Antibiotics for sore throat. *Cochrane Database Syst Rev.* 2013; (11).

145. Turck D, Bernet JP, Marx J, et al. Incidence and risk factors of oral antibiotic-associated diarrhea in an outpatient pediatric population. *J Pediatr Gastroenterol Nutr.* 2003;37(1):22-26.

146. Hirschhorn LR, Trnka Y, Onderdonk A, Lee M-LT, Platt R. Epidemiology of Community-Acquired Clostridium difficile-Associated Diarrhea. *J Infect Dis.* 1994;169(1):127-133.

147. Seckeler MD, Hoke TR. The worldwide epidemiology of acute rheumatic fever and rheumatic heart disease. *Clin Epidemiol.* 2011;3(1):67-84.

148. Matthys J, De Meyere M, Van Driel ML, De Sutter A. Differences among international pharyngitis guidelines: Not just academic. *Ann Fam Med.*

2007;5(5):436-443.

149. Little P, Stuart B, Richard Hobbs FD, et al.
Predictors of suppurative complications for acute
sore throat in primary care: Prospective clinical
cohort study. *BMJ.* 2013;347(November):1-14.

150. Yeh B, Eskin B. Should sore throats be treated with
antibiotics? *Ann Emerg Med.* 2005;45(1):82-84.

151. Mattu A, Martinez JP, Kelly BS. Modern
management of cardiogenic pulmonary edema.
Emerg Med Clin North Am. 2005;23(4):1105-1125.

152. Vasko JS, Henney RP, Oldham HN, Brawley RK,
Morrow AG. Mechanisms of action of morphine in
the treatment of experimental pulmonary edema.
Am J Cardiol. 1966;18(6):876-883.

153. Vismara LA, Leaman DM, Zelis R. The effects of
morphine on venous tone in patients with acute
pulmonary edema. *Circulation.*
1976;54(2):335-337.

154. Ellingsrud C, Agewall S. Morphine in the treatment
of acute pulmonary oedema--Why? *Int J Cardiol.*
2016;202(3):870-873.

155. Hoffman JR, Reynolds S. Comparison of
nitroglycerin, morphine and furosemide in
treatment of presumed pre-hospital pulmonary
edema. *Chest.* 1987;92(4):586-593.

156. Sacchetti A, Ramoska E, Moakes ME, McDermott

P, Moyer V. Effect of ED management on ICU use in acute pulmonary edema. *Am J Emerg Med.* 1999;17(6):571-574.

157. Peacock WF, Hollander JE, Diercks DB, Lopatin M, Fonarow G, Emerman CL. Morphine and outcomes in acute decompensated heart failure: an ADHERE analysis. *Emerg Med J.* 2008;25(4):205-209.

158. Miró Ò, Gil V, Martín-Sánchez FJ, et al. Morphine Use in the ED and Outcomes of Patients With Acute Heart Failure: A Propensity Score-Matching Analysis Based on the EAHFE Registry. *Chest.* 2017;152(4):821-832.

159. Wang K, Samai K. Role of high-dose intravenous nitrates in hypertensive acute heart failure. *Am J Emerg Med.* 2019;(xxxx):158324.

160. Shribman AJ, Smith G, Achola KJ. Cardiovascular and catecholamine responses to laryngoscopy with and without tracheal intubation. *Br J Anaesth.* 1987;59(3):295-299.

161. Derbyshire DR, Chmielewski A, Fell D, Vater M, Achola K, Smith G. Plasma catecholamine responses to tracheal intubation. *Br J Anaesth.* 1983;55(9):855-860.

162. White PF, Schlobohm RM, Pitts LH, Lindauer JM. A Randomized Study of Drugs for Preventing Increases in Intracranial Pressure during

Endotracheal Suctioning. *Anesthesiology.* 1982;57(3):242-244.

163. STEINHAUS JE, GASKIN L. A study of intravenous lidocaine as a suppressant of cough reflex. *Anesthesiology.* 24:285-290.

164. Poulton TJ, James FM. Cough suppression by lidocaine. *Anesthesiology.* 1979;50(5):470-472.

165. Bedford RF, Winn HR, Tyson G, Park TS, Jane JA. Lidocaine Prevents Increased ICP after Endotracheal Intubation. In: *Intracranial Pressure IV.* Berlin, Heidelberg: Springer Berlin Heidelberg; 1980:595-598.

166. Donegan MF, Bedford RF. Intravenously administered lidocaine prevents intracranial hypertension during endotracheal suctioning. *Anesthesiology.* 1980;52(6):516-518.

167. Bedford RF, Winn HR, Tyson G, Park TS, Jane JA. Lidocaine Prevents Increased ICP after Endotracheal Intubation. In: *Intracranial Pressure IV.* Berlin, Heidelberg: Springer Berlin Heidelberg; 1980:595-598.

168. Bedford RF, Persing JA, Pobereskin L, Butler A. Lidocaine or thiopental for rapid control of intracranial hypertension? *Anesth Analg.* 1980;59(6):435—437.

169. White PF, Schlobohm RM, Pitts LH, Lindauer JM. A

randomized study of drugs for preventing increases in intracranial pressure during endotracheal suctioning. *Anesthesiology*. 1982;57(3):242-244.

170. Guay J. Adverse events associated with intravenous regional anesthesia (Bier block): a systematic review of complications. *J Clin Anesth*. 2009;21(8):585-594.

171. Modica PA, Tempelhoff R. Intracranial pressure during induction of anaesthesia and tracheal intubation with etomidate-induced EEG burst suppression. *Can J Anaesth*. 1992;39(3):236-241.

172. Renou AM, Vernhiet J, Macrez P, et al. Cerebral blood flow and metabolism during etomidate anaesthesia in man. *Br J Anaesth*. 1978;50(10):1047-1051.

173. Dearden NM, Mcdowall DG. Comparison of etomidate and althesin in the reduction of increased intracranial pressure after head injury. *Br J Anaesth*. 1985;57(4):361-368.

174. Meikle J. Scanner scandal: are zoos using animal equipment on obese humans? The Guardian.

175. Kolata G. Why Do Obese Patients Get Worse Care? Many Doctors Don't See Past the Fat. *New York Times*. https://www.nytimes.com/2016/09/26/health/obese-patients-health-care.html. Published September 25, 2016.

176. Tello HCS, Cabodevila EM. Zooper Scanners Do Not Exist! Veterinarian Imaging Modalities Are Not An Option For The Morbidly Obese. :2786.

177. Ginde AA, Foianini A, Renner DM, Valley M, Camargo CA. The challenge of CT and MRI imaging of obese individuals who present to the emergency department: A national survey. *Obesity*. 2008;16(11):2549-2551.

178. Hawley PC, Hawley MP. Difficulties in diagnosing pulmonary embolism in the obese patient: A literature review. *Vasc Med*. 2011;16(6):444-451.

179. NICHOL ES, PHILLIPS WC, CASTEN GG. Virtue of prompt anticoagulant therapy in impending myocardial infarction: experiences with 318 patients during a 10-year period. *Ann Intern Med*. 1959;50(5):1158-1173.

180. Amsterdam EA, Wenger NK, Brindis RG, et al. 2014 AHA/ACC Guideline for the Management of Patients with Non-ST-Elevation Acute Coronary Syndromes: a report of the American College of Cardiology/American Heart Association Task Force on Practice Guidelines. *J Am Coll Cardiol*. 2014;64(24):e139-e228.

181. Niccoli G, Banning AP. Heparin dose during percutaneous coronary intervention: How low dare we go? *Heart*. 2002;88(4):331-334.

182. Cavender MA. Anticoagulants in Patients Undergoing PCI: Have New Data Made Heparin the Treatment of Choice?

183. Shahzad A, Kemp I, Mars C, et al. Unfractionated heparin versus bivalirudin in primary percutaneous coronary intervention (HEAT-PPCI): an open-label, single centre, randomised controlled trial. *Lancet (London, England).* 2014;384(9957):1849-1858.

184. Grüntzig AR, Senning A, Siegenthaler WE. Nonoperative dilatation of coronary-artery stenosis: percutaneous transluminal coronary angioplasty. *N Engl J Med.* 1979;301(2):61-68.

185. Topol EJ, Bonan R, Jewitt D, et al. Use of a direct antithrombin, hirulog, in place of heparin during coronary angioplasty. *Circulation.* 1993;87(5):1622-1629.

186. Grayburn PA, Willard JE, Brickner ME, Eichhorn EJ. In vivo thrombus formation on a guidewire during intravascular ultrasound imaging: evidence for inadequate heparinization. *Cathet Cardiovasc Diagn.* 1991;23(2):141-143.

187. Théroux P, Ouimet H, McCans J, et al. Aspirin, heparin, or both to treat acute unstable angina. *N Engl J Med.* 1988;319(17):1105-1111.

188. The Risk Group. Risk of myocardial infarction and death during treatment with low dose aspirin and

intravenous heparin in men with unstable coronary artery disease. The RISC Group. *Lancet (London, England).* 1990;336(8719):827-830.

189. Holdright D, Patel D, Cunningham D, et al. Comparison of the effect of heparin and aspirin versus aspirin alone on transient myocardial ischemia and in-hospital prognosis in patients with unstable angina. *J Am Coll Cardiol.* 1994;24(1):39-45.

190. Cohen M, Adams PC, Parry G, et al. Combination antithrombotic therapy in unstable rest angina and non-Q-wave infarction in nonprior aspirin users. Primary end points analysis from the ATACS trial. Antithrombotic Therapy in Acute Coronary Syndromes Research Group. *Circulation.* 1994;89(1):81-88.

191. Gurfinkel EP, Manos EJ, Mejaíl RI, et al. Low-molecular-weight heparin during instability in coronary artery disease, Fragmin during Instability in Coronary Artery Disease (FRISC) study group. Lancet (London, England).

192. Onwordi ENC, Gamal A, Zaman A. Anticoagulant Therapy for Acute Coronary Syndromes. *Interv Cardiol (London, England).* 2018;13(2):87-92.

193. Ribotsky BM, Berkowitz KD, Montague JR. Local anesthetics. Is there an advantage to mixing

solutions? *J Am Podiatr Med Assoc.*
1996;86(10):487-491.

194. Thomson CJ, Lalonde DH. Randomized double-blind comparison of duration of anesthesia among three commonly used agents in digital nerve block. *Plast Reconstr Surg.* 2006;118(2):429-432.

195. Ding R, Jung JJ, Kirsch TD, Levy F, McCarthy ML. Uncompleted emergency department care: patients who leave against medical advice. *Acad Emerg Med.* 2007;14(10):870-876.

196. Pennycook AG, McNaughton G, Hogg F. Irregular discharge against medical advice from the accident and emergency department--a cause for concern. *Arch Emerg Med.* 1992;9(2):230-238.

197. Alfandre DJ. "I'm going home": discharges against medical advice. *Mayo Clin Proc.* 2009;84(3):255-260.

198. Taqueti VR. Leaving against medical advice. *N Engl J Med.* 2007;357(3):213-215.

199. SMITH HW. LEGAL RESPONSIBILITY FOR MEDICAL MALPRACTICE. *J Am Med Assoc.* 1941;116(25):2755.

200. Levy F, Mareiniss DP, Iacovelli C. The importance of a proper against-medical-advice (AMA) discharge: how signing out AMA may create significant liability protection for providers. *J Emerg*

Med. 2012;43(3):516-520.

201. Monico EP, Schwartz I. Leaving against medical advice: facing the issue in the emergency department. *J Healthc Risk Manag.* 2009;29(2):6-9, 13, 15.

202. Kraut A, Fransoo R, Olafson K, Ramsey CD, Yogendran M, Garland A. A population-based analysis of leaving the hospital against medical advice: Incidence and associated variables. *BMC Health Serv Res.* 2013;13(1):1.

203. Alfandre D, Brenner J, Onukwugha E. Things We Do For No Reason: Against medical advice discharges. *J Hosp Med.* 2017;12(10):836-839.

204. Jerrard DA, Chasm RM. Patients leaving against medical advice (AMA) from the emergency department--disease prevalence and willingness to return. *J Emerg Med.* 2011;41(4):412-417.

205. Lekas H-M, Alfandre D, Gordon P, Harwood K, Yin MT. The role of patient-provider interactions: Using an accounts framework to explain hospital discharges against medical advice. *Soc Sci Med.* 2016;156:106-113.

206. Devitt PJ, Devitt AC, Dewan M. Does identifying a discharge as "against medical advice" confer legal protection? *J Fam Pract.* 2000;49(3):224-227.

207. Horwitz L, Lin Z, Grady J, et al. Hospital-Wide (All-

Condition) 30-Day Risk-Standardized Readmission Measure. *Yale New Haven Heal Serv Corp Outcomes Res Eval.* 2011;10.

208. Doenicke A. Etomidate, a new intravenous hypnotic. *Acta Anaesthesiol Belg.* 1974;25(3):307-315.

209. Chiu HH, Van WK. Clinical evaluation of etomidate as an induction agent. *Anaesth Intensive Care.* 1978;6(2):129-133.

210. Ledingham IM, Watt I. Influence of sedation on mortality in critically ill multiple trauma patients. *Lancet (London, England).* 1983;1(8336):1270.

211. Owen H, Spence AA. Etomidate. *Br J Anaesth.* 1984;56(6):555-557.

212. Fragen RJ, Shanks CA, Molteni A, Avram MJ. Effects of etomidate on hormonal responses to surgical stress. *Anesthesiology.* 1984;61(6):652-656.

213. Abraham E, Evans T. Corticosteroids and septic shock. *J Am Med Assoc.* 2002;288(7):886-887.

214. Absalom A, Pledger D, Kong A. Adrenocortical function in critically ill patients 24 h after a single dose of etomidate. *Anaesthesia.* 1999;54(9):861-867.

215. Annane D, Sébille V, Charpentier C, et al. Effect of treatment with low doses of hydrocortisone and

fludrocortisone on mortality in patients with septic shock. *JAMA*. 2002;288(7):862-871.

216. Zed PJ, Mabasa VH, Slavik RS, Abu-Laban RB. Etomidate for rapid sequence intubation in the emergency department: is adrenal suppression a concern? *CJEM*. 2006;8(5):347-350.

217. Lipiner-Friedman D, Sprung CL, Laterre PF, et al. Adrenal function in sepsis: The retrospective Corticus cohort study. *Crit Care Med*. 2007;35(4):1012-1018.

218. Ray DC, McKeown DW. Effect of induction agent on vasopressor and steroid use, and outcome in patients with septic shock. *Crit Care*. 2007;11(3):1-8.

219. Riché FC, Boutron CM, Valleur P, et al. Adrenal response in patients with septic shock of abdominal origin: Relationship to survival. *Intensive Care Med*. 2007;33(10):1761-1766.

220. Schenarts CL, Burton JH, Riker RR. Adrenocortical dysfunction following etomidate induction in emergency department patients. *Acad Emerg Med*. 2001;8(1):1-7.

221. Hildreth AN, Mejia VA, Maxwell RA, Smith PW, Dart BW, Barker DE. Adrenal suppression following a single dose of etomidate for rapid sequence induction: A prospective randomized study. *J*

Trauma - Inj Infect Crit Care. 2008;65(3):573-578.

222. Upchurch CP, Grijalva CG, Russ S, et al. Comparison of Etomidate and Ketamine for Induction During Rapid Sequence Intubation of Adult Trauma Patients. *Ann Emerg Med.* 2017;69(1):24-33.e2.

223. Price K, Allen U, Mandersloot G, Shirley P, McAuley D. Effect of a single dose of etomidate on adrenal function in patients with trauma. *Crit Care 2005; 9.* 2005;9:S163–4. 6.

224. Den Brinker M, Hokken-Koelega ACS, Hazelzet JA, De Jong FH, Hop WCJ, Joosten KFM. One single dose of etomidate negatively influences adrenocortical performance for at least 24 h in children with meningococcal sepsis. *Intensive Care Med.* 2008;34(1):163-168.

225. Jones AE, Yiannibas V, Johnson C, Kline JA. Emergency department hypotension predicts suddden unexpected in-hospital mortality: A prospective cohort study. *Chest.* 2006;130(4):941-946.

226. Franklin C, Samuel J, Hu TC. Life-threatening hypotension associated with emergency intubation and the initiation of mechanical ventilation. *Am J Emerg Med.* 1994;12(4):425-428.

Made in the USA
Monee, IL
09 August 2023

40663611R00061